Fatness, Obesity, and Disadvantage in the Australian Suburbs

Megan Warin • Tanya Zivkovic

Fatness, Obesity, and Disadvantage in the Australian Suburbs

Unpalatable Politics

palgrave
macmillan

Megan Warin
University of Adelaide
Adelaide, SA, Australia

Tanya Zivkovic
University of Adelaide
Adelaide, SA, Australia

Disclaimer: This views expressed in this publication do not necessarily reflect South Australian Government policies.

ISBN 978-3-030-01008-9 ISBN 978-3-030-01009-6 (eBook)
https://doi.org/10.1007/978-3-030-01009-6

Library of Congress Control Number: 2019931005

Cover image: MBI / Alamy Stock Photo
Cover design: Fatima Jamadar

This Palgrave Macmillan imprint is published by the registered company Springer Nature Switzerland AG.
The registered company address is: Gewerbestrasse 11, 6330 Cham, Switzerland

Preface: Apples—Toffee Apples—Toffs

Apples have long been associated with all manner of symbols and mythology. From religious contexts (the forbidden fruit in the Garden of Eden) to the byte/bite from the Apple logo, apples are rich with meaning. In the obesity debate, the apple frequently appears as a symbol of good health. The old adage "an apple a day keeps the doctor away" is a popular saying believed to originate from the 1860s in Wales. Green and red apples are ubiquitous images in corporate health advertising and public health promotions. Often circled with a tape measure or stethoscope, the message is clear and simple—that eating an apple is good for your waistline, and for your health.

Apples can also be transformed into other edible delights, most famously the sugar-coated toffee apple depicted on the cover of this book, a treat that one might find sold at showgrounds or fairs. Viewed as confectionery, the healthy, fresh apple is dipped in boiled sugar syrup, which has been colored red and allowed to set, before being wrapped in cellophane. The apple is now transformed into a sugary delight on a stick, a gift of sweetness that resembles a lollipop more than an apple. Once the sugary syrup is gone, most of the apple is thrown away, as the apple is no longer so desirable.

Toffee also has connotations beyond the taste of sweetness. Toffee has been transformed and wrapped in class-based ideology. The English expression "toffee-nosed" means "posh" and is then shortened to the colloquial "toff." The term toff was recorded by Henry Mayhew in *London Labour and the London Poor* (1851), as a name given by the lower classes in Victorian England to stylishly dressed upper-class gentlemen. In our

Australian fieldwork "toffee" was used by working-class people to describe those "who were sort of posh and people who talked down to us." Far removed from the pleasures of sugary toffee that can be dissolved in mouths, toffee here is inserted into vernacular representations of hierarchy and class.

Food and health—never as simple as we assume.

Adelaide, SA, Australia

Megan Warin
Tanya Zivkovic

Acknowledgments

This book is the culmination of many years of research and conversations. We are grateful to the Australian Research Council for funding the project (LP 120100155), and to the external partners who also contributed funds and support in kind. Michelle Jones was instrumental in facilitating this partnership, and we thank her for her support and guidance in navigating these relationships. We would like to thank Vivienne Moore and Paul Ward for their intellectual engagement with the project, and their sustained commitment to putting forward the marginalized narratives that were central to this work. We would also like to extend our gratitude to the external partners involved, in particular the Obesity Prevention and Lifestyle (OPAL) staff. There were points of disagreement along the way, and we are mindful of the challenges that working in this field of obesity prevention hold. It is not an easy space in which to make changes. Other community members played a role in supporting the project, and we extend thanks to Ken Daniels, who brought his extraordinary clarity to the project and insight into the politics of local government. Ruthie O'Reilly provided wonderful research assistance, and we thank her for her meticulous attention to the interview material.

Many departmental colleagues and national and international audiences have provided important feedback regarding questions of ethnographic detail and theoretical insight, and we are grateful for the capacity to think with such scholars. Special thanks to Stanley Ulijaszek, Amy McLennan, Michelle Pentecost, Karin Eli, Elisabeth Hsu, and members of the Unit for Biocultural Variation for Obesity in the Institute of Social and Cultural Anthropology at the University of Oxford who provided a platform to discuss our research over the years. Thanks also to Lynne Giles, Jessie Gunson, Wendy Wills, Lucy Farrell, John Coveney, Teresa Davis, Christopher Mayes, Michael Davies, Jackie Street, Bridget Jay, Erica Millar, the Life Course and Intergenerational Health Research Group, and Food Values Research Group at the University of Adelaide, and members of the Australian Food, Society and Culture Network, who all gave feedback on the project at differing times. Special thanks to Freya Barr and Valerie Mobley for their meticulous editing skills, and to the University of Adelaide's Research Branch (Simon Brennan and Oana Monale) who provided expert advice at key points of the research. We were delighted to work with Palgrave Macmillan and offer our appreciation to Alexis Nelson and Kyra Saniewski, who have helped steer this work to fruition. We especially thank Mary Al-Sayed for her care and patience in this process.

Most importantly, we wish to thank all the community members who were involved in the research. Without their time, generosity, and willingness to share their lives, this book would not be possible.

Contents

Abbreviations

ABC	Australian Broadcasting Corporation
ABS	Australian Bureau of Statistics
ADG	Australian Dietary Guidelines
AGHE	Australian Guide to Healthy Eating
ANPHA	Australian National Preventive Health Agency
ARC	Australian Research Council
BMI	Body mass index
CBD	Central Business District
CHD	Coronary heart disease
COAG	Council of Australian Governments
EPODE	Ensemble Prévenons l'Obésité des Enfants
GMH	General Motors Holden
HAES	Health at Every Size
NCMP	National Child Measurement Programme
NPAPH	National Partnership Agreement on Preventive Health
OPAL	Obesity Prevention and Lifestyle
PNNS	Programme National Nutrition Santé
SAHT	South Australian Housing Trust
SBS	Special Broadcasting Service
SES	Socioeconomic status
SIMPLA	Stop Income Management in Playford
SPAG	Single Parents Action Group
TAFE	Technical and Further Education
UNESCO	United Nations Educational, Scientific and Cultural Organization
WHO	World Health Organization

List of Figures

CHAPTER 1

Introduction

In May 2015 Australia's independent broadcaster, Special Broadcasting Service (SBS), released a promotional video of a three-part documentary called *Struggle Street*. The show depicted families living in Sydney's outer-western suburbs, an area well recognized as experiencing significant socio-economic hardship. The promotional video began with upbeat music and a deep-toned, male voice-over, contrasting the glistening waters and tanned, lithe, bikini bodies of Sydney Harbor and beaches with the graffitied, litter-strewn, and drug-taking lives of people living on the fringes. The video caused a great stir among Australia's media and the local mayor complained that the show misrepresented his residents. There was an immediate flurry, involving lawyers, accusations of defamation, and an online petition demanding the television program be stopped from airing. A protest by garbage truck drivers from Sydney's west was staged outside the SBS studios, with the mayor proclaiming, "The program is garbage so we've brought garbage trucks out here as a symbolic protest. This is a false representation [of Blacktown] and this program must stop."

Despite the protests, the three shows went to air, although staged quickly over one week, rather than the planned three weeks. Given this frenzied and high-profile prelude, the viewing audience was huge, and many commentators applauded the ways in which the documentary sensitively portrayed the families, their strong sense of pride, and resilience in the face of adversity. Others, however, said it copied TV shows in the UK

M. Warin, T. Zivkovic, *Fatness, Obesity, and Disadvantage in the Australian Suburbs*,
https://doi.org/10.1007/978-3-030-01009-6_1

(such as the BBC's *Benefits Street*, set in Northern England), where Middlesbrough football fans protested against the show by unfurling a banner at the club's Riverside Stadium, which read "Being Poor Is Not Entertainment—Fuck Benefits Street" (Tyler 2015). Such protests argue that these types of reality shows are nothing more than "poverty porn," exploiting vulnerable people to increase ratings and denigrate those living on welfare benefits.

The very same week, we gave a presentation to university colleagues on our research into how a community with high levels of disadvantage responded to Australia's largest childhood obesity intervention. Specifically, this ethnographic project explored how people living in what the state's Department of Health refers to as an "obesogenic environment" (Government of South Australia, Annual Report 2008–2009) understood risk and why they displayed resistance to public health imperatives. Tanya described the significant economic downturn of the area since the 1970s, and the health issues that all too frequently accompany chronic unemployment, high rates of mental illness, and precarious lives. She didn't show pictures of our research participants' houses (as that would be unethical), but she did show houses that were typical of the area in which our fieldwork was located. She shared stories of how research participants resisted moralized stereotypes of obesity through humor, pushing back against neoliberal "responsibilization" by appropriating the word "fat" and its many euphemisms as a form of joking or endearment. Questions from the audience were mixed, with suggestions that the representations were inaccurate, misrepresentative, or biased in their selection. Someone asked if we'd seen *Struggle Street*, again making an implicit accusation and clear analogy to the reproduction of "poverty porn."

While *Struggle Street* and our ethnographic project are entirely different, there are some startling similarities to the politics of representation and positioning that each brings to light. Our research encountered a similar range of applause and accusation, of "telling it like it is" and misrepresenting the community. As Emma Kowal's work on white antiracism in Australia showed, any discussion of sensitive issues, like class or race, the portrayal of Aboriginal Australians, or whiteness involves an "endless potential for misinterpretation" (2015, p. 24). When we talked about obesity in relation to social class, we also encountered an endless and inescapable potential for misinterpretation. So much so that after the first year of our three-year research project, Tanya lamented that she could not return to her field site of India (where her ethnographic focus was on death and reincarnation), as it was nowhere near as political as researching obesity in Australia!

This book is about the politics of fat. It tells the story of what happens when a French childhood obesity intervention is purchased by the Australian Government and implemented in one of Australia's most disadvantaged suburban communities. On the face of it, obesity prevention appears to be straightforward, simply encouraging and educating people on how to make healthy lifestyle choices, to eat healthier foods, and increase physical activity. But of course it's not so simple. For families who have very limited incomes, scraping a few cents together to buy bare essentials or to ask for out-of-date bread from the local food bank is a regular reality. Being told to choose more healthy options is unrealistic when their choices are already severely constrained and parents are looking for something filling and cheap to fill empty stomachs. Messages to eat less when your body aches from hunger seem incongruent with everyday realities. For women who use the flesh of their bodies to "get things," being told to lose weight threatens their local economy of trading sexuality for drinks at the local club. And for people in the community who are well aware of the shame of obesity and the common stereotypes of living in a disadvantaged community, being targeted for being fat or incapable of looking after themselves is seen by many as just another assault on their self-esteem.

The story that unfolds in this book has a dual purpose. It firstly exposes the complex politics involved in Australia's largest obesity prevention campaign, from the government health bureaucrats, the public health nutritionists and dieticians, the local government workers, the social marketing team, and the anthropologists researching the program (us) to the people who are the target of such a program—people who live precarious lives where "getting by" frequently takes precedence over healthy eating. As anthropologists working in the community, we learned about how locals resisted healthy eating initiatives, rejected middle-class imperatives of healthy living, and crafted their own stories around health and fatness.

We also learned of the various hierarchies and conflicts within the community, and the various moral views about how people should work and demonstrate citizenship in the community. Many of the participants in our project were on welfare benefits, volunteering through a federal Australian Government "mutual obligation" scheme to comply with welfare payment policies and surviving on very limited incomes. At the height of punishing South Australian summer heat waves, some people said that their fans and air conditioners were too expensive to switch on, leading to sometimes dire consequences for the very young or the elderly residents in public housing. Some could not afford to shower every day due to expensive water bills, and some houses did not have fridges, with one participant using a camp stove in her kitchen as it was cheaper to run than her oven and cooktop. Pride and shame circulated in equal measure in this community, and unsurprisingly (as others have similarly noted (Shildrick et al. 2010; Shildrich and MacDonald 2013)), in a depressed economy a process of "Othering" and distancing occurs, where people can be outright disparaging of those who are still more disenfranchised than they are.

Secondly, the book provides a timely analysis of the relationships between differing kinds of knowledge about obesity. We explore the many tensions and misunderstandings that arise within partnerships of anthropology, public health, and local government: of the devaluing of ethnographic research methods as unrepresentative, of the unpalatability of bringing critiques or frames of social class into our analysis, and of the attempts to silence or alter research findings. We were quickly reminded that all knowledge projects are political, and one can never be free from the values and interests of particular social locations (Kirksey 2011, p. 157). Our research inevitably entered the political game of representation, encountering the stakes involved in positive and positivist research outcomes. We would become aware of who can say what, of which words and voices are silenced, and of multiple contested knowledges, representations, and portrayals of people, health, and poverty.

As many commentators have noted, obesity is an intensely political issue, and this book deals with the machinations of local government power structures, assumptions of "willful ignorance," and class-based politics. This work contributes to a growing number of ethnographic studies of obesity, including Yates-Doerr's long-term fieldwork in Guatemala (Yates-Doerr 2015a), Solomon's work on metabolism and obesity in India (Solomon 2016), McLennan and Hardin's research on the Melanesian Islands of Nauru and Samoa (Hardin 2015; McLennan 2013), and Popenoe's work on gender and fatness in Niger (Popenoe 2004). Our work differs from these ethnographies as it is situated in our home city and focused directly on a community that was the target of the state's largest childhood obesity intervention. This provided us with a unique fieldwork opportunity to examine the politics of an obesity intervention as it unfolded, working not only with the staff of the statewide public health team and local council, but also with people and places in the community.

Ethnographic methods and anthropological critique were unsettling for some, particularly for those in positions of power who were not accustomed to "studying up" or working with the messiness of ethnographic data.

In an era where many anthropologists do work in the health arena to provide critical engagement with public health problems, such as obesity (Warin et al. 2015, 2017; Yates-Doerr 2015a), food insecurity (Carney 2015), HIV/AIDS (Human immunodeficiency virus/Acquired immune deficiency syndrome; Eves 2012; Jordan Smith 2014; Nguyen 2010; Reynolds-Whyte 2014), Ebola (Nguyen 2014), dengue fever and Zika (Nading 2014, 2015), smoking (Dennis 2016), and so on, politics is centrally placed—the politics around knowledge, resources, and the power to determine what is rational or not in terms of understandings, behaviors, and practices. This book thus critically examines the politics of obesity research—of how obesity interventions are done in practice—and also the politics of academic and bureaucratic engagement.

It is not often that the politics of research partnerships are openly talked about.[1] In a precarious funding environment for research, it is with good reason that researchers might wish to gloss over conflict and simply present narratives that talk of positive findings. In 2015 the *Medical Journal of Australia* published an article about university health research, suppression, and open enquiry. The authors reported on a survey conducted in 2006 with Australian public health researchers, which found that 21% of respondents experienced a funding-related suppression event—something that sanitized, delayed, or prohibited the publication of research findings (Kypri 2015, p. 72). Not surprisingly, the respondents said their work was targeted because they drew attention to the failing of health services and/or the health status of a vulnerable group. There are very few discussions in the academic literature of how these external relationships unfold. From our experiences and anecdotal discussions with social science colleagues working on public health issues, both nationally and internationally, we are aware of how years of research data can be suppressed and/or destroyed by government or industry partners, or where research results are simply blocked from publication or dissemination. Researchers, however, tend not to write about failures of this kind for fear of retribution or reputational damage.

In seeking to understand these points of conflict, we draw upon the work of many scholars from differing fields: anthropologists, sociologists, science and technology studies scholars, feminists, and social geographers, exploring the ways in which obesity is constructed (Guthman 2013; Ulijaszek 2017) and enacted (Mol 2002; Yates-Doerr 2015a). Firstly, we look to the ways in which dominant positionings of obesity foreclose critical analysis and reproduce narrow understandings of "the problem." Emilia Sanabria's work on the social production of ignorance within the field of public health nutrition in France extends this argument, suggesting that there is a tendency in obesity interventions to rely on established idioms and ways of thinking (2016, p. 135). We demonstrate the difficulties of opening up alternative modes of knowing "the problem," and the ways in which academic research is drawn into fields of evidence that have already been structured by these relations (Sanabria 2016, p. 154).

In Ingold's (2017) *Knowing from the Inside*, he writes: "Sometimes one's best ideas come not from following the main lines of an investigation but from veering off course, in brief encounters with things … and people that trigger reflections on quite unfamiliar and unexpected topics" (2017, p. 4). This is how we approached obesity as a topic of research, looking for different ways to think beyond the taken-for-granted constraints of problem closure. Annemarie Mol (2002) takes a similar line in her philosophical discussion of atherosclerosis, offering a relational and practice-oriented approach to her study of the multiple realities of how this disease is "done" in practice. She chose to do this as she was dissatisfied with the social science separation of disease and illness—with how the study of the disease itself (and the physical body) was left to physicians, opening the way for discursive interpretations of culturally specific meanings of bodies. It is as if the object of study, be it atherosclerosis or fat, could be placed, like an object "in the middle of a circle," and different epistemological viewpoints of the "thing" could be presented and critiqued by "medical doctors, nurses, technicians, patients, or whoever else is concerned" (Mol 2002, p. 12). This has meant that social scientists have marked the space of illness meanings and experiences as their turf, and "granted biomedicine the exclusive right to talk about the body and its diseases" (Mol 2002, p. 13). The result is a chasm between these different types of knowledges, in which "one point of view differs from that of another" (ibid.), and often there is no space for conversation or collaboration between these differences.

In *The Body Multiple* (2002), Mol urges us to take another step and foreground the practicalities, materialities, and events of the disease in question, to explore how, in our case, obesity becomes a part of what occurs in practice. It is this line of inquiry that we have attempted to follow in this book, to make visible the situations and relations in which fatness and eating are performed, rather than situate obesity as a fixed and inert thing. Obesity and fat leak across and into different domains, enabling multiple realities depending on what people are doing and in what situation. We seek a more widespread understanding of these multiple fatnesses.

An Ethnographic Study of Risk and Resistance

Between 2012 and 2015 we led a team of academic researchers on an ethnographic project investigating how a community in the northern suburbs of Adelaide, South Australia, responded to Australia's largest childhood obesity program. The public health intervention was called Obesity Prevention and Lifestyle (OPAL) program and had significant federal, state, and local government investment of A$40 million over a 10-year period of 2008–2018 (OPAL Collective 2015, p. 375). The program was based on a French franchise (Ensemble Prévenons l'Obésité des Enfants [EPODE]), and South Australia was the first state in the southern hemisphere to run this initiative. OPAL's overall goal was to "improve eating and activity patterns of children, through families and communities in OPAL regions, and thereby increase the proportion of 0–18 year-olds in the healthy weight range" (ibid., p. 376). Guided by a "logic model," OPAL's conceptual framework was based on three different theories: socioecology, social marketing, and community development (OPAL Collective 2015, p. 376).

OPAL focused on educating the community, particularly children and families, about the importance of good health and healthy eating. In aiming to change lifestyle behaviors, OPAL's social marketing team "identified specific behaviors that were seen as unhealthy and formulated specific themes to encourage behavior change." These themes were taken up at local government level and worked on in conjunction with a community well-being initiative. Examples of these behavior changes included well-intentioned public health messages, such as "nudging" people to drink water rather than soft drinks, to walk, ride a bicycle or scooter to school rather than get a lift in a car, and turn off screens and play outside. A range of social marketing messages were distributed in the community by way of brochures, banners, marketing items (such as branded Frisbees, breakfast bowls, and water bottles), and educational sessions were presented at schools, local community centers, childcare centers, and kindergartens.

The first phase of the OPAL program began in 2009 and was initiated in six communities.[2] Many of the first-stage locations had areas which were described by OPAL as "doing it tough" and having "multiple disadvantages whereby one social problem is compounded by other problems" (Baum et al. 2005). The program was expanded across several timed phases to include 21 different communities.

The academic research team included two anthropologists (the authors of this book), two senior public health academics (trained in sociology and social epidemiology), as well as the OPAL evaluation manager who worked in the SA State Government (and had a background in social sciences). Our research was a researcher-initiated competitive grant scheme funded by the federal Australian Government. As a group we had extensive experience in health-related research (including obesity), in working with external partners, and in ethnographic research. Our two industry partners included a state government health department located in a security-conscious high-rise building in the heart of the city and the local council of the area involved in the program. Across our external partners we worked with a range of people and health professionals, including the state manager of the OPAL program, a council-appointed manager of the OPAL program, project officers working for or in partnership with OPAL, council food bank staff and volunteers, and a number of community development managers and social marketing officers. Throughout the life of the project there was a frequent turnover of local government and food bank staff (due to job losses and frequent restructures in local government), which often resulted in new staff being brought in to comment on our findings along the way.

At the time of applying for the grant, it was well documented that treatment and prevention initiatives for obesity were largely ineffective (Thomas 2006; Thomas et al. 2010; Walls et al. 2011). Australian Government initiatives were calling for more innovative ways to tackle the "obesity problem" (Seear et al. 2010) and the need to identify the broader contextual features (social, cultural, political, and economic) of obesity (Seear et al. 2010). We claimed that there was little knowledge about everyday understandings of obesity, or about how public health messages on obesity were received by different groups (including those from different socioeconomic groups).

In linking in with OPAL, we sought to investigate how families from low socioeconomic communities responded to obesity interventions. In particular, the project aimed to explore how the community understood risks associated with obesity (if at all), and if gender and social class intersected to influence responses to obesity intervention strategies. We explicitly wanted to identify points of uptake and resistance to the obesity interventions that OPAL was introducing to the community, and anticipated that project outcomes would provide key insights to inform obesity policy and prevention strategies that were responsive to local realities of risk and resistance.

The Study Area

The ethnographic site for our study was situated approximately 30 km north of the Adelaide CBD (central business district) in the City of Playford council area. This site is diverse in terms of population (approximately 92,000 residents) but "when compared to all local government areas in the Adelaide Statistical Division, is ranked as the most disadvantaged area in metropolitan Adelaide" (City of Playford 2008) and one of the most disadvantaged urban areas in Australia (Hordacre et al. 2013). A third of households live in poverty and there is a high incidence of unemployment and underemployment (Hordacre et al. 2013). As comparative studies in low- and high-income areas of Adelaide show, low-income families spend a higher proportion of their income on food and this is constrained by other household expenses (including the rising costs in housing and utilities), leading therefore to a greater prevalence of "food stress" (Ward et al. 2013; Wong et al. 2011). Most families in our study conveyed that healthy foods were outside their purchasing power and, as a result, cheaper foods, which tend to be higher in fat or sugar, become more enticing out of a "taste of necessity" (Bourdieu 1984).

In this community there are significant levels of housing stress, financial and food insecurity, psychological distress, substance dependence, and self-rated poor health (Burns 2014; City of Playford 2008; Hordacre et al. 2013). During fieldwork Tanya was surprised when, on her first day in the field, there was a robbery at the shopping center where she was volunteering. It wasn't just the robbery per se that shocked her, but the nonchalance of the workers who did not react to this drama, and simply kept on about their business as if this was part and parcel of everyday routines (Fig. 1.1).

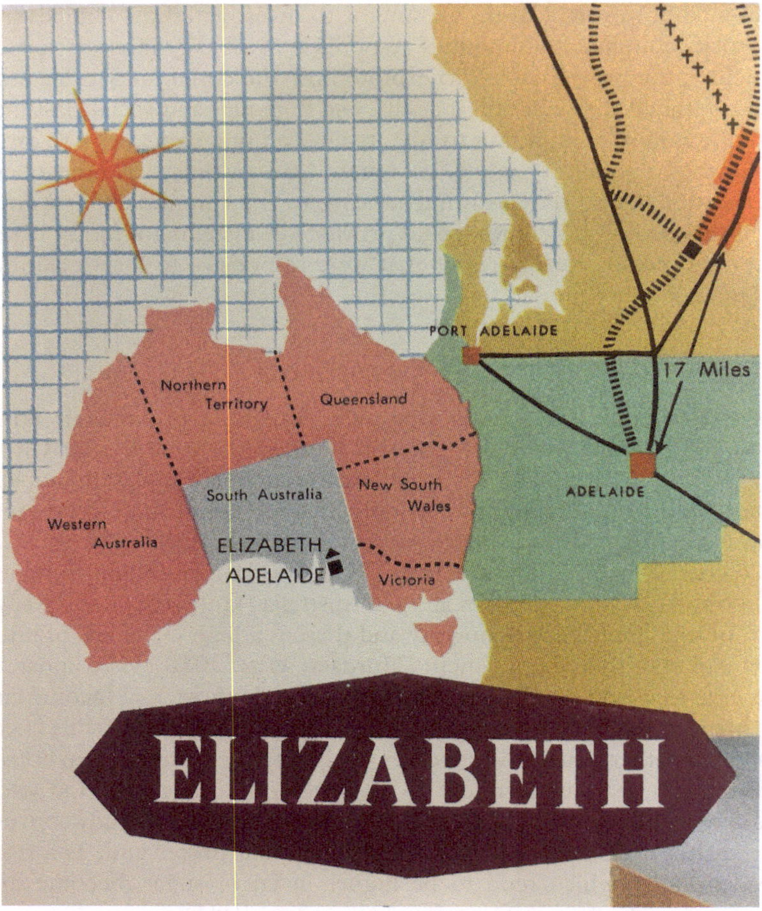

Fig. 1.1 A 1959 South Australian Housing Trust brochure depicting the location of Elizabeth "Build your future in Elizabeth: a prosperous city in a rapidly expanding state … South Australia." (Dates/Publication details: Adelaide: South Australian Housing Trust, 1959)

While not explicitly named as an obesogenic environment by the OPAL team, our study locale could be characterized as such (Swinburn et al. 1999). The concept of the obesogenic environment is based on the theory that people are obese because they "are surrounded by cheap, fast, nutritionally inferior food [and live in] a built environment that discourages physical activity" (Guthman 2013, p. 142). The model then assumes that people are more likely to have an increased energy intake of less nutritious foods and beverages but limited physical output, thus resulting in higher rates of obesity (Public Health Information Development Unit 2013, p. 16). OPAL also had a clear mandate for improving the infrastructure of the local environment and worked in partnership with local government to improve health-enhancing facilities (e.g. walkways, playgrounds). It was because a problem of overweight and obesity had been identified in this community that the proactive local government (City of Playford), seeking solutions, welcomed OPAL into the community.

While some participants in our study spoke of a strong community pride that comes from facing continuing hardship and austerity, they acknowledged the many social problems (domestic violence, unemployment, food insecurity, and mental illness) that have become embedded across generations and need to be faced on a day-to-day basis. This was made even more pressing by the continuing uncertainty around General Motors Holden (GMH), which discontinued all operations in Australia in October 2017. Car manufacturing had been a central feature of the local workforce and identity ever since the original suburb of Playford (Elizabeth) was laid out in the 1950s, and participants often talked about the detrimental impact that this loss of jobs and industry focus would have on their community. In this context of such employment insecurity it is not difficult to understand that survival or "getting by" takes priority, thus helping to explain why lower adherence to healthy eating guidelines is consistently reported in less affluent areas (Bambra et al. 2012; Warin et al. 2015).

Our investigation method was ethnographic, and we conducted participant observation and in-depth interviews with people living and working in the community as well as semi-structured interviews with key stakeholders in the OPAL program. Data collection occurred over a period of 23 months (August 2012–July 2014), during which time the principal ethnographer (Tanya) was located in the broader community and at two food bank locations (where she volunteered for 14 months), and another researcher conducted the majority of face-to-face interviews with 37 families and 10 stakeholders involved with OPAL (including community workers, local government employees, and state government managers). Most interviewees (varying in age from 18 to 65) were of Anglo-Saxon heritage, and seven interviewees identified as Indigenous Australians. Some of our fieldwork encounters were with local migrant communities (East African and South East Asian), a growing demographic of recent arrivals in the area.

We explored taken-for-granted understandings of food, bodies, and activity, and sought to identify whether obesity interventions might encounter strong cultural resistance to perceived social change. Tanya was provided with office space in the council "operations center," a building protected by a barbed wire fence that housed local government workers. We caught trains and buses to and from, and within the field; we volunteered in food banks; we walked through neighborhoods to meet and spend time with people in their own homes; we accessed local community services; and we waited at train stations, sat in food courts, and shopped in local stores.

Two food banks provided a window into members of the community who were down on their luck. These community food banks have been established for two decades and stock cheap foods, meal packs, household items, like nappies and basic toiletries, and a small selection of fruit and vegetables. When first set up in the 1990s they were a pilot program explicitly aimed at addressing food insecurity and intended to last for six months. A long-standing volunteer described how they sold limited and very basic items: "the cheapest possible options—one brand of baked beans and tinned spaghetti." Meal packs (dinners to be made at home) were supplied for Aboriginal families through a local Indigenous health service and sold at very low prices. To the volunteers' surprise, the food bank pilot program kept going. One of the current managers explained: "The people wanted it and so it was successful" (Fig. 1.2).

Roles in our fieldwork were highly gendered, reflecting the dominance of women in the food service industry, in nutrition and dietetics, the public health workforce in healthy weight and food, and the central role that women continue to play in household and family food and eating. The majority of participants we interviewed were young women with caring responsibilities. Of the two community men we interviewed, one described himself as a "house mum." Shoppers in the food banks were often women (mainly young mothers), with the next group dominated by older single men. All but one of the paid workers in the food banks were women, as were most of the volunteers. As the government welfare scheme required recipients to volunteer, it was not surprising that people opted for volun-

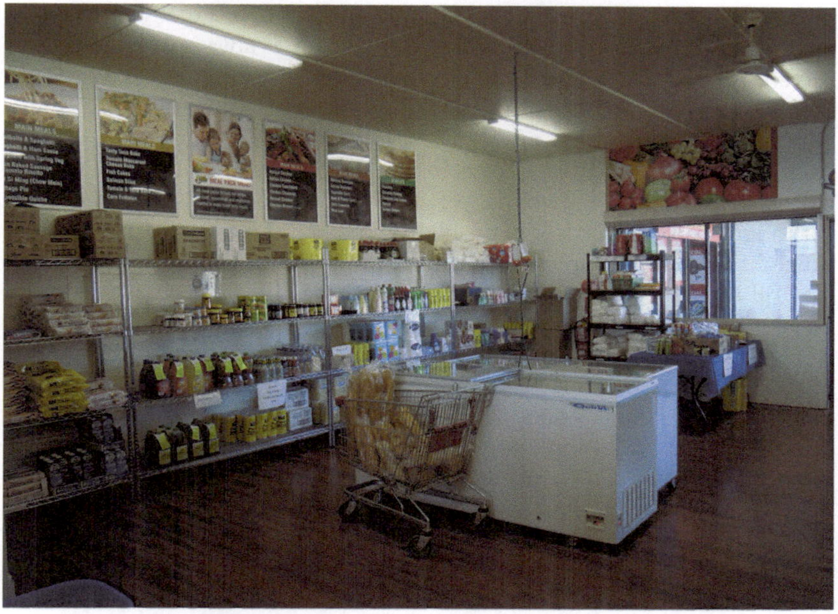

Fig. 1.2 One of the food banks in our fieldwork location. (Photo from Authors)

teering roles in which they already had skills; women opted for volunteering roles in the food and service sector, and men for driving roles.

Food banks played important caring roles in each community. These were places where people could not only find affordable foods, but also ask for help with problems. The coordinator at each site was a woman who lived in the community and had intimate knowledge of everyday struggles. Along with all the volunteers they were familiar with and empathized with people's circumstances. One site was known to sometimes "bend the rules a little," helping people with free food, connecting with others, and offering a shoulder to lean on. Workers described the food banks as "family," where they shared commensality each day over lunch, snacks, and laughter, pleased with the perks of cheap and free food.

Days in the food bank had their own rhythm. The doors opened at 9:30 a.m., and after morning greetings and cups of instant coffee, there were decisions about tasks, and anticipation of lunch. Mornings were usually dedicated to preparing meal packs, dividing foods (white sugar, frozen hash browns, bags of grated cheese) into smaller parcels to sell, and stocking shelves. Tanya is told on her first day: “There is always work to do and this sort of preparation will help us when it comes to the next big order or the next busy period of customers. Now, have you had your lunch?” Tanya says she has eaten. “The other girls are having their lunch now out the back. Leonie and I will have ours in a minute when they’re finished. It is better to always have two people at the front of the shop. It’s safer. Although we’ve never had a problem here, for the most part. The post office has been held up as have other shops around here. So come with me, I’ll introduce you to the other ladies here and show you where you can put your bag to keep it safe.”

As described in Garthwaite’s (2016) ethnographic study of food banks in the North of England, the food bank volunteers pared back items to make them affordable—shoppers could buy one egg, instant coffee divided into small bags, or a single toilet roll. Members of the community could come in with coins in their hand (and frequently did so). Not long after Tanya started work in one of the food banks, she noticed a young woman paying for her goods with a handful of coins retrieved from the bottom of a handbag and Vivienne,[3] the volunteer staff member, having to take the coins out the back to wash them. This excerpt from fieldwork observations with the volunteer staff at the food bank describes the incident:

> *The money that Vivienne [a food bank volunteer] had been given was a handful of 5-cent pieces and they were covered in greenish blue ink which the woman had tried to clean, leaving the coins quite damp. Katie [another food bank worker] tells me, “This woman, she’s come in a number of times. She tends to come in when she is literally down to her last pennies, when she’s only a few cents left. … We try our best with these people to give them something to tide them over until more money comes in, to give them something to make a meal with, like we can sell an egg or two and give them some bread—now that might just be enough to get them through or to feed their children before they get paid tomorrow.”*

We learned (like Garthwaite 2016) that the reasons why people use food banks are complex. Not surprisingly, life circumstances that result in ill-health, unemployment, and disability were key factors in bringing people through these doors.

The Perils of Invoking Neoliberalism

During our research we had regular meetings with our external partners to update them on our findings. In addition, we were called to several meetings to talk about findings that OPAL staff found "unpalatable." The first related to a Foucauldian analysis of the social marketing campaign that encouraged people to eat breakfast—not just any breakfast but "a healthy breakfast" (Warin et al. 2017) that was promoted to children as "brain food." We drew on theoretical work to examine the ways in which the purchase and consumption of high-fiber breakfast cereals and other foods (e.g. wholegrain foods for "wholegrain goodness") were embedded in historical, religious, and nutritional discourses about the moral fiber of persons. Such discourses, we argued, underscore assumptions about the proper temporal order for day-to-day family life, in which parents are urged to regulate the bodies of themselves and their children in time and in space—in what Coveney referred to as the "nutritional homescape" (2006, p. 107). Training sessions, which we attended for the OPAL staff at a state government education center, confirmed these discourses, as preparing and eating breakfast was clearly promoted as "a proxy for general levels of organization." Governance occurs across differing levels of persons, families, and peristaltic movements, intertwining to keep family time and also bodies regular, disciplined, and punctual.

We argued that the social marketing of a healthy breakfast overlooks aspects of the wider sociocultural context in which people live in a community. When local service providers were introduced to the breakfast social marketing theme, a case manager from an agency responsible for managing unemployment benefits said she liked the idea, but wondered how she could actually translate this meaningfully to local families: "Many families do not have food in the cupboard every day of the week. They are struggling financially in the lead-up to payday. They're grappling with drug and alcohol addictions, serious mental health issues, and traumatic life histories" (Warin et al. 2017, p. 223). Healthy breakfasts are clearly not part of everyone's everyday ***habitus*** and are out of reach for many households.

We were called into the offices of the state's health department to account for our interpretation and analysis of the data. On a whiteboard a series of dot points were written, inviting us to articulate what our project was "really about," to explain what ethnography was, whether we had consent from all participants, and how we could claim that the project was representative (not that we did claim this). There was implied distrust and skepticism about the perceived lack of objectivity in an embodied and immersive ethnographic study (c.f. Holmes 2006). Our hearts sank as we immediately recognized the devaluing of qualitative research, because "what counts [in obesity interventions] is largely determined by the possibility of demonstrating the efficacy of intervention numerically" (Sanabria and Yates-Doerr 2015, p. 118).[4] We put forward explanations about the conduct of ethnographic research and attending to specificities (rather than representativeness), and the rigor of this approach. This was difficult, as arguing for particular situations and concerns, and showing how these were shaped by multiple, coexistent, and at times ambivalent and contradictory contingencies, was met with puzzled expressions (Sanabria and Yates-Doerr 2015, p. 122). These sorts of explanations could not be neatly "scaled up."

In coming up against what Bell and Green (2016) refer to as "the perils of invoking neoliberalism" in public health critique, we were essentially being asked to defend and legitimize the methodological and theoretical premise of the project. Moreover, there were tight media controls from the external partners concerning potentially negative press releases concerning OPAL, to the point where our work was deemed to be "too risky" to be in the public sphere. This was an ongoing issue and one OPAL worker confided to us that some managers were more concerned about "protecting the brand of OPAL" even to the extent of blocking our publications, rather than seeing how our findings might help make adjustments and improvements to the program.

It is important to highlight that our perceptions of tensions in the project with our external partners were not with individuals or particular personalities. We believe that every OPAL worker came into the program with the intention of improving people's health and doing this in a sensitive way without stigmatizing the community. This is unquestionable. Rather, the tensions we highlight point to much bigger challenges which university–external relationships can entail. Our external partners were constrained by their own bureaucratic and political needs, and throughout the project it became increasingly evident that any critique was viewed as criticism and was not welcome. OPAL was already under intense public scrutiny and as we did not work for local or state government there were fears that we could not be controlled. Most importantly for the project as a whole was that OPAL appeared to have been implemented with a solution in mind (weight reduction among younger community members) before our project was even under way. Thus the table was already set and perhaps there was no place mat for anthropological knowledge that questioned, unsettled, or challenged. Receptivity to diverse forms of knowledge and engagements in debates that academics are familiar with is only useful to decision makers *before* problems have been determined, and not as part of the process. We reflect on these broader questions throughout the book, hoping to highlight some of the key tensions for academics engaged in future external partnerships.

The Distaste of Class

As well as the problems that arose when we highlighted the workings of biopower in health promotion discourses, others ensued when we were asked to present participants (their lives and narratives) in "more palatable" ways. We were often asked to remove photographs from our academic presentations that depicted class or historical change in the community. We were asked to remove an image of a postcard from an international conference presentation that promoted the township of Elizabeth in the 1950s as "Beautiful." The souvenir postcard sported "images of clean, angular factory buildings surrounded by gardens and the neat rectangles of car parks and flower beds" (Peel 1995, p. 64), and other newly built civic amenities such as the hospital, high school, the town shopping center, and a skating rink. Quotes from participants who spoke in a negative light about their neighborhood were similarly asked to be removed. These fieldwork images and words that depicted local realities were said to "promote a class distinction" and to be a "put down of people living in the area."

At one meeting about a third of the way through our project we were asked by an OPAL manager: "What's class got to do with it anyway?" We suddenly realized that the very notion of class to our research partners was distasteful, that the very mention of it could be viewed as a slur rather than an opportunity to expose inequality. Our research was premised on analyzing obesity and associated interventions in the context of class, recognizing that the term "social class" is a key structural determinant in health inequalities research. Class theory in relation to food, eating, and tasting bodies (encapsulated in Bourdieu's concepts of *habitus*, capital, and distinction) was central to our grant proposal. We reflected on why the word "class" was regarded by some of our external partners as unpalatable and even irrelevant: we came to realize that class is seen as a distasteful notion as it conveys prejudice against particular social groups. The local council followed "a strengths-based approach" to community issues and had an ongoing investment in dis-identifying with and distancing themselves from any kind of negative identity. Clearly, any association with negative representations or language was going to be highly problematic.

Identity politics was therefore used in a number of ways as a rationale for a requirement to paint positive stories of resilience and upward mobility. While we also dislike deficit models of people, we did not want to shy away from exposing inequalities. We would not whitewash or romanticize people's everyday experiences, and we pressed the point that acknowledging and understanding hardship and poverty was crucial to health promotion in this area. Later on, when we took our findings back to participants to check their responses to these representations, one long-term resident said "there are a lot of problems in Playford—you can't hide that."

While there are differing uses of the term "social class," Valentine and Harris (2014) argue that the category of class has become increasingly obscured in a climate where the "twin forces of individualization and de-traditionalization [have] emphasized the plasticity of individuals' identities and life chances" (2014, p. 84). Class has become an individual attribute (c.f. Krieger et al. 1997) in which social inequalities are reduced to individual stratification indicators, such as education (Muntaner et al. 2015). This neoliberal trend, which demonizes people for poor choices (poor food choices) and lack of self-management (poor bodily discipline) resonates with dominant models of the rational individual, rather than viewing peoples' circumstances through the lens of structural disadvantage (Valentine and Harris 2014, p. 86). In reflecting on his use of social distinctions and class relations between fictional characters, Australian author Tim Winton notes the awkward silences that the seemingly provocative ire of class gives rise to. In line with academic thought on social class and health inequities, Winton notes with sadness (and irony) that despite the rapid growth of inequality in Australian society in the last two decades, "Australians have been trained to remain uncharacteristically silent about the origins of social disparity" (Winton 2013).

While some managers and OPAL staff held a view that class was not relevant or should not be highlighted, many OPAL team members did "recognize the evidence that people 'at risk' of becoming overweight or obese are more likely to come from disadvantaged backgrounds" (OPAL Collective 2015, p. 379). It was clear to us from our fieldwork experiences and many conversations with OPAL staff in local communities that structural issues such as access and affordability were seen as important, but *less so* than the relational processes in which socioeconomic disparities were perpetuated.

Chapter-by-Chapter Outline

In Chap. 2 we explore the reasons why obesity is such a contentious and political issue in contemporary life. We trace the differing fields (in Bourdieu's sense) of who has the power to define obesity (as a disease, a lifestyle, a health risk) and the counter-narratives to this medical discourse. Rather than focusing on obesity as an object of study, social scientists (including anthropologists, sociologists, feminists) and fat activists have been highly critical of this medicalization and have challenged the pathologization of fatness and the rise of neoliberal imperatives of individual responsibility for health (Kwan and Graves 2013). This is symbolized in the rejection of the very word obesity, and a preference for the descriptor of "fat," as seen in the academic field of "fat studies." A recent call for papers for a Fat Studies conference requested that "submitters rethink using words like 'obesity' and 'overweight' in their presentations unless they are used ironically, within quotes, or accompanied by a political analysis."[5] Such a strategy aims to reclaim the language of bodies from pathological and medical gazes (Wann 2009, p. xiii). For most OPAL workers, seeing "obesity" in quotes—as a problematized category—just made no sense.

How you come to *know* obesity or fatness matters. We discovered early on that there were different sets of information for stakeholders and for OPAL communities. We asked Kellie, one of the OPAL social marketers (and herself a large woman) if the word obesity ever appeared in any of the materials for the community. She responded promptly:

> *Never. The word obesity is there in material for the stakeholders but it has never been in the material for community members. The two lots of material are really very separate. We never wanted the word obesity in there. For us it has always been about promoting healthy living in the community, people just do not identify with obesity.*

Already this thing called obesity shifts and slides in and out of view and is both present, yet absent. People understand obesity and its stigmatizing power in very different ways.

In Chap. 3 we introduce the reader to the global and local connections of the obesity program, and set the scene of the field site, the actors, and the ethnographic research process. The Australian obesity model is a direct franchise from the French-designed, community-based anti-obesity EPODE program (Ensemble, Prévenons l'Obésité des Enfants/Together Let's Prevent Childhood Obesity), which started in 1992 in two small towns (Fleurbaix and Laventie) in the north of France. EPODE is funded through international corporations such as Mars®, Nestlé®, Schweppes®, and Coca Cola®, and frames obesity as a problem of excessive eating and limited physical activity. Thus the standard "eat less and exercise more" mantra is at the heart of this prevention program. We describe how EPODE was transformed into the Australian model of OPAL, with an emphasis on a socio-ecological model and social marketing. OPAL was launched in Adelaide with great fanfare and enthusiasm, and despite the establishment of OPAL in a disadvantaged community with higher than average rates of overweight and obesity and the need for food banks, there was no mention of hunger or poverty.

Another time when we were called to a meeting with OPAL staff to discuss our draft publication of fat as productive (Zivkovic et al. 2018), we were asked where we live, as a covert way of marking class and establishing authority for who can speak. Two of the research team spent childhoods in similar neighborhoods of economic deprivation in the UK and Australia, with one, Tanya, having a biography intimately connected to the field site at which we were working. Members of the research team were perceived at different times (and by different people) as insiders and outsiders and we were always mindful that the function of drawing these types of boundaries was concerned with power and control.

As with all research, this book tells a partial story. Historian and academic, Professor Mark Peel has written several books on his own upbringing in Elizabeth (*Good Times, Hard Times: The Past and Future in Elizabeth* (1995); *The Lowest Rung: Voices of Australian Poverty* (2003)) in which he looks back to this intimacy of experience and textual representation:

> *Generalization is a hazardous business … there are obvious dangers in speaking of your own place: I must be wary of romanticizing, of nostalgia and self-justification masquerading as history, or of simply celebrating the Elizabeth I knew. … I must wonder if memory is "evidence" and how often and when I should use it. Certainly, I cannot speak for everyone. The story I tell is partial and it is probably at odds with the Elizabeth's other people remember.* (Peel 1995, p. 6)

Whether or not one is doing fieldwork "at home" or in places of unfamiliarity, ethnographic representations are always situated as "partial"

(Abu-Lughod 2008; Haraway 2003) and would never claim to represent all people.

There is a common belief both in academia and in popular discourse that poor people are fat because they don't know how to cook and lack nutritional knowledge. This "information deficit" model is dominant in public health interventions (Kowal 2015; Warin 2018; Yates-Doerr 2015a) and as a consequence it is thought that what is needed is up-skilling in nutritional knowledge and cooking skills. Ingold (2013) refers to this type of information as already "prepackaged," as it is authoritative knowledge that takes for granted the premise on which it is based. The very fact that OPAL started in a community that is well known for its disadvantage points to the implicit belief that nutritional education is needed to solve the obesity problem. Chapter 4 examines the ideological underpinnings of the OPAL program, and the ways in which nutritional discourse is "black-boxed" (Sanabria 2016; Scrinis 2013; Yates-Doerr 2012, 2013) when presented to the community. Implicit in this model is the neoliberal assumption that individuals can take responsibility for their nutritional intake and can make behavioral changes to improve their eating habits (Mayes 2016). We argue that prepackaged knowledge dismisses complexity (Sanabria 2016; Ulijaszek 2015), for the messy, contested, and contradictory nature of everyday lives is impossible to map.

In OPAL's approach to food, eating, and weight loss, certain components of foods were targeted: sugar, salt, and fat. The OPAL program presented sugar as a hidden danger and always sought to reduce people's sugar consumption. This policing of sugar content in drinks and foods caused consternation, as many participants used the pleasure and exchange of sugar as a form of everyday care and sociality. Chapter 5 examines the ways in which sugar sweetened relationships, and the greater value placed on relationships than health. When resources are limited, moments of pleasure become fewer and hence more valued. Volunteers in the food bank did not like OPAL's denial of pleasure; nor did they like to be "told they are doing it wrong … no one likes to be told what to eat."

As Michel de Certeau describes in *The Practice of Everyday Life* (1984), people in disempowered situations find cracks in which to "slip and slide" and to resist authority and filch back power. In the local food banks we witnessed the scramble to hide chocolates when OPAL staff were known to be coming, and the sneaking of salt into OPAL-prescribed foods that were bland and tasteless to local palates. Resistance to the dominant model of obesity as a medical calamity was also part of everyday discourses, where humor about each other's body sizes and the use of non-pathologized vernacular were common.

Chapter 6 interrogates the different versions of fat that are central to any obesity prevention campaign. Using ethnographic work from around the globe, we look at how large bodies are culturally sanctioned in many cultures, and fat is experienced as a positive attribute of personhood and relatedness. However, when we compare meanings of fat in Western health-related contexts we find that fatness is uniformly presented as negative. Our fieldwork participants, however, spoke of positive aspects of being fat, either as a way to distance the stigma and shame that was projected onto them or to use fatness as a means to "get stuff," and to shield them from the austerity of their everyday lives. In this neighborhood, thinness revealed the "hard knocks" of life in the haggard bodies of people with long-term drug addictions and those with severe mental illness. As a marker of socioeconomic disadvantage, thinness did not readily fit into gendered and classed values of fitness, beauty, and health. Interestingly, it was this work on the value of fatness that caused the most controversy with our government partners, who could not even conceive of fat being a positive attribute.

In our fieldwork the OPAL workers sometimes asked us: "Well, what would *you* do? What's *your* solution?" We always resisted answering simple questions with simple solutions, but in Chap. 7 we describe the many local practices of creativity that were central to de-stigmatization strategies. A major stumbling block in this type of population intervention was the power imbalance created by experts brought in to "bring people up to a certain level." Well-intentioned programs had the effect of pushing local knowledge aside, ignoring the many examples of what Mol calls "tinkering" (2010; Mol et al. 2010)—of how families and households "tinkered" with what was to hand in response to practices of care on limited incomes. This tinkering was often an enactment of pride, a counterbalance to the shame that so often permeated everyday encounters around fatness, hunger, and poverty. In our fieldwork one woman described herself as the "local Jamie Oliver," quizzing elderly people in her extended family who had been through the Great Depression and garnering tips about how to eat on a shoestring. This network of coping practices was an established part of the community fabric, but was not leveraged by the OPAL program.

The conclusion explores how ethnographic analysis has the potential to reorientate the ways we think about fatness and obesity. Anthropology does much more than provide a comprehensive picture of local knowledge. Anthropological techniques examine the very premise of the problems we research and can reframe and reposition the ways in which problems are understood. Obesity and obesity intervention programs cannot simply be scaled up or scaled down, from the global to the local. Scaling, as anthropologists Anna Tsing (2012) and Emily Yates-Doerr (2015b) argue, erases difference and assumes objects (in this case obesity and eating) to be fixed and stable categories that can be transported from and across local, national, and global sites. Importantly, this book provides a narrative to help those implementing obesity programs to open the possibility that fatness and obesity have multiple, coexistent realities. In unraveling the story of our anthropological research and the many frictions we encountered, this work is also a timely caution about how anthropologists might work with any number of health or government professionals who take explanations of obesity for granted.

Notes

1. David Mosse (2005), Eben Kirksey (2011), and Emma Kowal (2015) discuss the difficulties of accountability and interpretation they encountered during their ethnographic fieldwork. Employed as an anthropologist-consultant on a British aid development project in rural India, Mosse describes the rupture of relationships he encountered. He details how different actors responded to his analysis—it was "accepted and challenged, endorsed and dismissed, recognised and unrecognised; it has intrigued and depressed, provoked incandescence and been utterly ignored" (2005, p. 14).
2. In all, there were 21 communities involved in OPAL across South Australia, including one community in the Northern Territory (referred to as the Childhood Obesity Prevention and Lifestyle [COPAL] program).
3. Pseudonyms have been used for all research participants and in some cases roles and place names have been changed to further protect anonymity.
4. Rail et al. (2010) make a similar observation when they argue that obesity science relies on "a process that is saturated by ideology and intolerance regarding certain types of evidence, alternative discourses, and non-normative knowledge and ways of knowing (for example, qualitative research)" (Rail et al. 2010, p. 262).
5. https://fattitudethemovie.files.wordpress.com/2015/10/cfp-fsnz2016.pdf Conf on Fat Studies 2016.

References

Abu-Lughod, L. (2008). Writing against culture. In T. Oakes & P. L. Price (Eds.), *The cultural geography reader* (pp. 62–71). London: Routledge.

Bambra, C., Hillier, F., Moore, H., & Summerbell, C. (2012). Tackling inequalities in obesity: A protocol for a systematic review of the effectiveness of public health interventions at reducing socioeconomic inequalities in obesity amongst children. *Systematic Reviews, 1*, 16.

Baum, S., O'Connor, K., & Stimson, R. (2005). *Fault lines exposed: Advantage and disadvantage across Australia's settlement system.* Monash University Press. Retrieved from http://books.publishing.monash.edu/apps/bookworm/view/Fault+Lines+Exposed%3A+Advantage+and+Disadvantage+Across+Australia%E2%80%99s+Settlement+System/138/xhtml/copyright.html

Bell, K., & Green, J. (2016). On the perils of invoking neoliberalism in public health critique. *Critical Public Health, 26*(3), 239–243.

Bourdieu, P. (1984). *Distinction: A social critique of the judgment of taste* (trans: Nice, R.). Cambridge: Harvard University Press.

Burns, J. (2014). The human cost of the shifting economy: Holden's closure and Elizabeth's future. *Australian and New Zealand Journal of Psychiatry, 48*(4), 375–376.

Carney, M. A. (2015). *Unending hunger.* Oakland: University of California Press.

City of Playford. (2008). *Poverty and low income, Community Wellbeing Plan (2006–2011).* https://www.playford.sa.gov.au/webdata/resources/files/Poverty_and_Low_Income_Fact_Sheet_June_2007.PDF

Coveney, J. (2006). *Food, morals and meaning: The pleasure and anxiety of eating* (2nd ed.). London: Routledge.

De Certeau, M. D. (1984). *The practice of everyday life.* Berkeley: University of California Press.

Dennis, S. (2016). *Smokefree: A social, moral and political atmosphere.* London: Bloomsbury Publishing.

Eves, R. (2012). Resisting global AIDS knowledges: Born-again Christian narratives of the epidemic from Papua New Guinea. *Medical Anthropology, 31*(1), 61–76.

Garthwaite, K. (2016). *Hunger pains: Life inside foodbank Britain.* Bristol: Policy Press.

Government of South Australia. (2009). *Department of Health Annual Report 2008–2009.* Adelaide. https://tinyurl.com/yd7kkw3s

Guthman, J. (2013). Too much food and too little sidewalk? Problematizing the obesogenic environment thesis. *Environment and Planning, 45*(1), 142–158.

Haraway, D. (2003). Situated knowledges: The science question in feminism and the privilege of partial perspective. *Turning Points in Qualitative Research: Tying Knots in a Handkerchief, 2003*, 21–46.

Hardin, J. (2015). Christianity, fat talk, and Samoan pastors: Rethinking the fat-positive-fat-stigma framework. *Fat Studies, 4*(2), 178–196.

Holmes, M. (2006). Review of the book *Blush: faces of shame*, by E. Probyn (2005). *Body & Society, 12*(1), 123–126.

Hordacre, A. L., Spoehr, J., Crossman, S., & Barbaro, B. (2013). *City of Playford: Socio-demographic, employment and education profile.* Adelaide: Australian Workplace Innovation and Social Research Centre.

Ingold, T. (2013). Foreword. *Education in the North, 20* (Special issue) 1. Retrieved from https://www.abdn.ac.uk/eitn/documents/Volume%2020%20Special%20Issue/EITN%20Volume%2020%20foreword.pdf

Ingold, T. (2017). *Knowing from the inside.* Aberdeen: University of Aberdeen.

Jordan Smith, D. (2014). *AIDS doesn't show its face: Inequality, morality, and social change in Nigeria.* Chicago: University of Chicago Press.

Kirksey, S. E. (2011). Don't use your data as a pillow. In A. Waterston & M. Vesperi (Eds.), *Anthropology off the shelf: Anthropologists on writing* (pp. 146–159). Oxford: Blackwell.

Kowal, E. (2015). *Trapped in the gap: Doing good in Indigenous Australia.* Oxford: Berghahn Press.

Krieger, N., Williams, D., & Moss, N. (1997). Measuring social class in US public health research: Concepts, methodologies, and guidelines. *Annual Review of Public Health, 18*(1), 341–378.

Kwan, S., & Graves, J. (2013). *Framing fat: Competing constructions in contemporary culture.* New Brunswick: Rutgers University Press.

Kypri, K. (2015). Suppression clauses in university health research: Case study of an Australian government contract negotiation. *The Medical Journal of Australia, 203*(2), 72–74.

Mayes, C. (2016). *The biopolitics of lifestyle: Foucault, ethics and healthy choices.* New York: Routledge.

McLennan, A. (2013). *An ethnographic investigation of lifestyle change: Living for the moment, and obesity emergence in Nauru.* Unpublished PhD thesis, University of Oxford.

Mol, A. (2002). *The body multiple: Ontology in medical practice.* Durham: Duke University Press.

Mol, A. (2010). Care and its values: Good food in the nursing home. In A. Mol et al. (Eds.), *Care in practice: On tinkering in clinics, homes and farms* (pp. 215–234). New London: Transaction Publishers.

Mol, A., Moser, I., & Pols, J. (2010). *Care in practice: On tinkering in clinics, homes and farms.* New London: Transaction Publishers.

Mosse, D. (2005). *Cultivating development: An ethnography of aid policy and practice.* London: Pluto Press.

Muntaner, C., Ng, E., Chung, H., & Prins, S. J. (2015). Two decades of Neo-Marxist class analysis and health inequalities: A critical reconstruction. *Social Theory & Health, 13*(3–4), 267–287.

Nading, A. (2014). *Mosquito trails: Ecology, health and the politics of entanglement.* Oakland: University of California Press.

Nading, A. (2015). The lively ethics of global health GMOs: The case of the oxitec mosquito. *BioSocieties, 10*, 24–47.

Nguyen, V. K. (2010). *The republic of therapy: Triage and sovereignty in West Africa's time of AIDS.* Durham: Duke University Press.

Nguyen, V. K. (2014, October 7). Ebola: How we became unprepared, and what might come next. *Cultural Anthropology Online.* Retrieved from http://www.culanth.org/fieldsights/605-ebola-how-we-became-unprepared-and-what-might-come-next

OPAL Collective. (2015). Practitioner insights on obesity prevention: The voice of South Australian OPAL workers. *Health Promotion International, 31*(2), 375–384.

Peel, M. (1995). *Good times, hard times: The past and the future in Elizabeth.* Carlton: Melbourne University Press.

Peel, M. (2003). *The lowest rung: Voices of Australian poverty.* Cambridge: Cambridge University Press.

PHIDU – Public Health Information Development Unit. (2013). *Public Health Information Development Unit, The University of Adelaide.* Accessed from: http://www.lga.sa.gov.au/webdata/resources/files/Playford-1.pdf

Popenoe, R. (2004). *Feeding desire: Fatness, beauty and sexuality among a Saharan people.* London: Routledge.

Rail, G., Holmes, D., & Murray, S. J. (2010). The politics of evidence on 'domestic terrorists': Obesity discourses and their effects. *Social Theory & Health, 8*(3), 259–279.

Reynolds Whyte, S. (2014). *Second chances: Surviving AIDS in Uganda.* Durham: Duke University Press.

Sanabria, E. (2016). Circulating ignorance: Complexity and agnogenesis in the obesity 'epidemic. *Cultural Anthropology, 31*(1), 131–158.

Sanabria, E., & Yates-Doerr, E. (2015). Alimentary uncertainties: From contested evidence to policy. *BioSocieties, 10*, 117–124.

Scrinis, G. (2013). *Nutritionism: The science and politics of dietary advice.* New York: Columbia University Press.

Seear, K., Fraser, S., Wright, J., Maher J., & Petersen, A. (2010). Peeling away the onion. *Report on a National Consultation on childhood obesity research, policy and practice in Australia.* Centre for Women's Studies and Gender Research, Monash University.

Shildrich, T., & MacDonald, R. (2013). Poverty talk: How people experiencing poverty deny their poverty and why they blame the poor. *The Sociological Review, 61*(2), 286–303.

Shildrick, T., MacDonald, R., Webster, C., & Garthwaite, K. (2010). *The low-pay, no-pay cycle*. York: Joseph Rowntree Foundation.

Solomon, H. (2016). *Metabolic living: Food, fat, and the absorption of illness in India*. Durham: Duke University Press.

Swinburn, B., Egger, G., & Raza, F. (1999). Dissecting obesogenic environments: The development and application of a framework for identifying and prioritizing environmental interventions for obesity. *Preventive Medicine, 29*(6), 563–570.

Thomas, H. (2006). Obesity prevention programs for children and youth: Why are their results so modest? *Health Education Research, 21*(6), 783–795.

Thomas, S., Lewis, S., Hyde, J., Castle, D., & Komesaroff, P. (2010). The solution needs to be complex: Obese adults' attitudes about the effectiveness of individual and population based interventions for obesity. *BMC Public Health, 10*, 420.

Tsing, A. (2012). On nonscalability: The living world is not amenable to precision-nested scales. *Common Knowledge, 18*(3), 505–524.

Tyler, I. (2015). Classificatory struggles: Class, culture and inequality in neoliberal times. *The Sociological Review, 63*, 493–511.

Ulijaszek, S. (2015). With the benefit of foresight: Reframing the obesity problem as a complex system. *BioSocieties, 10*(2), 213–228.

Ulijaszek, S. J. (2017). *Models of obesity: From ecology to complexity in science and policy*. Cambridge: Cambridge University Press.

Valentine, G., & Harris, C. (2014). Strivers vs skivers: Class prejudice and the demonisation of dependency in everyday life. *Geoforum, 53*, 84–92.

Walls, H., Peeters, A., Proietto, J., & McNeil, J. (2011). Public health campaigns and obesity: A critique. *BMC Public Health, 11*(1), 136.

Wann, M. (2009). *The fat studies reader*. New York: New York University Press.

Ward, P. R., Verity, F., Carter, P., Tsourtos, G., Coveney, J., & Wong, K. C. (2013). Food stress in Adelaide: The relationship between low income and the affordability of healthy food. *Journal of Environmental and Public Health, 2013*. [online]. Retrieved from http://www.hindawi.com/journals/jeph. https://doi.org/10.1155/2013/968078.

Warin, M. (2018). Information is not knowledge: Cooking and eating as skilled practice in Australian obesity education. *The Australian Journal of Anthropology, 29*(1), 108–124.

Warin, M., Zivkovic, T., Moore, V., Ward, P. R., & Jones, M. (2015). Short horizons and obesity futures: Disjunctures between public health interventions and everyday temporalities. *Social Science & Medicine, 128*, 309–315.

Warin, M., Zivkovic, T., Moore, V., & Ward, P. (2017). Moral fibre: Breakfast as a symbol of a 'good start' in an Australian obesity intervention. *Medical Anthropology: Cross-Cultural Studies in Health and Illness, 36*, 217. https://doi.org/10.1080/01459740.2016.1209752.

Winton, T. (2013, December). The C word: Some thoughts about class in Australia. *The Monthly*, 24.

Wong, K. C., Coveney, J., Ward, P., Muller, R., Carter, P., Verity, F., & Tsourtos, G. (2011). Availability, affordability and quality of a healthy food basket in Adelaide, South Australia. *Nutrition and Dietetics, 68*(1), 8–14.

Yates-Doerr, E. (2012). The opacity of reduction: Nutritional black-boxing and the meanings of nourishment. *Food, Culture and Society, 15*(2), 293–313.

Yates-Doerr, E. (2013). Complex carbohydrates: On the relevance of ethnography in nutrition education. In E. J. Abbots & A. Lavis (Eds.), *Why we eat, how we eat: Contemporary encounters between foods and bodies* (pp. 271–287). Farnham: Ashgate.

Yates-Doerr, E. (2015a). *The weight of obesity: Hunger and global health in postwar Guatemala*. Berkeley: University of California Press.

Yates-Doerr, E. (2015b). Intervals of confidence: Uncertain accounts of global hunger. *BioSocieties, 10*(2), 229–246.

Zivkovic, T., Warin, M., Moore, V., Ward, P., & Jones, M. (2018). Fat as productive: Enactments of fat in an Australian suburb. *Medical Anthropology: Cross Cultural Studies in Health and Illness, 37*(5), 373–386.

CHAPTER 2

Why Is Obesity Such a Political Issue?

Can You Be Fat and Healthy?

In 2013, during the course of our research, an Australian television documentary series (*Insight*) broadcast a program on obesity called *Fat Fighters*. The series is known for airing topical and controversial issues in a debate-style format and aims to present all sides of the story. The small audience of about 25 people sat on tiered seats and was peppered with a range of "experts," as well as people who would be considered obese according to the body mass index (BMI) scale. There was a small stage for three guests, and the moderator was a well-respected female journalist (Jenny Brockie) who asked questions and moderated discussion between the guests and the audience. The program immediately started with a question from the moderator to a guest on the stage. "Dorothy, describe your body for me." Dorothy casually replied: "Curvy, voluptuous, carefree, and just big and beautiful." Dorothy was a large Pacific Islander woman who said she loved her body and that it was "ideal" for a Samoan woman. Asked how she'd be viewed if she were thinner, she said with some incredulity that people would think she was sick. Some members of the audience laughed at this incongruous remark—knowing that in Australian society it is fat people who are deemed unwell, not thin people. The presenter turned to the audience and asked a different woman, Karen, how her body was viewed in Australia. Karen was a large white woman with a slash of red matte lipstick, who said that there was a perception that being big was associated

M. Warin, T. Zivkovic, *Fatness, Obesity, and Disadvantage in the Australian Suburbs*,
https://doi.org/10.1007/978-3-030-01009-6_2

with being unhealthy, undesirable, and gluttonous. She spoke of growing up and feeling shame and disgust from self-directed fat phobia and the "cruel optimism" (Berlant 2011) of 20 years of diet failures. Karen is an academic from an Australian university who focuses on fat phobia, feminism, and fat bodies.

The next question was raised by a fresh-faced young man who was a fitness trainer, and he politely started with: "[I]t's great that people can be any size they want." But then he asked Karen if she had been to a doctor to check if she was healthy. Karen shot an eye-rolling glance back as she responded angrily: "That's a loaded question, and anyone here who is thin is not going to be asked that question. … I do think there is such a health focus in this country … you can't tell someone's lifestyle or health just by looking at them … there's such a moral obligation for people to be ***healthy*** in this country!" Acting the provocateur, Jenny kept coaxing: "But isn't that because it costs taxpayers a lot of money? If the population isn't healthy, people have to go to hospital and they have various kinds of diseases." A middle-aged man piped up to say there was too much focus on discrimination and we should focus on the health aspects for everybody. "Being fat," he said, in a matter-of-fact tone, "is not good for the individual; it's not good for society and certainly not good for the health dollar. The medical system is buckling under the sheer weight of the 60% of people who are overweight and obese." The audience laughed uneasily at his unintended pun.

The debate continued and more people were drawn in to give their points of view: a public health academic spoke about the population risk of obesity; a clinical psychologist who worked with people who had body image problems and eating disorders; refugees and migrants from Africa who have experienced nutritional transitions and put on weight (and developed diabetes) after arriving in Australia; a general practitioner and academic who worked with migrant communities; a bariatric surgeon and a mother and daughter who had both had bariatric surgery; and a woman who took matters into her own hands and had cut a swathe of fleshy fat from her own body.

The last ten minutes of the show dissolved into an argument between a large woman in the audience and a thin female fitness trainer. A question that conflated health with fatness was directly targeted at a large woman in the back row and came with an accusatory tone: "Are you healthy? What do you eat?" The woman (wearing a whale badge—a symbol of fat activists) steadfastly refused to answer, standing her ground against the moral imperative implied in such a question. She stated that this type of question (and the whole discussion) "is very indicative of the prevailing attitude toward fatness [negative and morally loaded] … and the refusal to accept that there can be other ways of living."

What this episode of *Fat Fighters* presented was a clear example of what has become known as "the obesity wars." Whoever you are, your gender, your cultural identification, your political persuasion, your own body size, your training in life sciences, social sciences, or humanities—people will disagree on whether being fat is unhealthy, whether large bodies are culturally beautiful or signal a lack of self-care, and whether individuals should be held accountable and responsible for the economic burdens of body size. Food and eating also hold different values—is food functional (eaten for health) or experienced as expressions of care and comfort? What is "food for rich people" and does eating "white man's food" signal success back home for migrants? Each position is shot through with moral judgments about personhood, and, of course, one's own body size and identity politics have major roles to play. Gender, class, race, and epistemological training are all platforms for positioning different stances in relation to fat, and the one who had the power or privilege to speak was not always equal.

What this tells us is that obesity is not simply one thing.[1] In this chapter we explore the tensions that *Fat Fighters* presents, as these are key themes in the book. There is no escaping that popular narratives that classically construct obesity as a discursive problem, through the power of statistics and quantifiable metrics (McCullough and Hardin 2013; Yates-Doerr 2013), appeal to economic imperatives, and our fear of the harms of disease. This is the underpinning rationale of the Obesity Prevention and Lifestyle (OPAL) program. But as we learned from our fieldwork and *Fat Fighters*, people don't always agree about how problems are constructed and foreclosed, and a raft of alternative ways of knowing and being fat exist. Contestations and conflicts ensue between these different Bourdieurian fields, as players struggle for legitimacy, authority, and a voice. It is not our intention to say who is right or wrong or to pitch these debates in fragmented pieces. Our intention, and drawing on Mol (2002) for this inspiration, is to investigate the multiple versions of fatness and obesity, and the ways in which they are enacted.

The Rise (and Plateauing) of Obesity

It is undeniable that overweight and obesity is now presented as a significant global problem. Twitter feeds, public media, and academic journals are crammed with stories and facts and figures about rising levels of obesity, with dire warnings that our children will be the first generation to die younger than their parents due to risks associated with being overweight or obese. A 2016 study from *The Lancet* on global trends in adult BMI across 200 countries has been converted into a dynamic visualization of "the contagious way that obesity has spread virally around the world" (NCD Risk Factor Collaboration 2016). The map moves across time and allows viewers to watch "how the world got fat" from 1975 to 2014. The darker the color a country becomes, the fatter its adult population has become, and 200 countries in this graphic change to a deeper color.

The map no longer presents obesity as the "curse of the western world," since it is now found in countries that have historically (and still) experience malnutrition or famine. The World Health Organization (WHO) acknowledges that "once considered a problem only in high-income countries, overweight and obesity are now dramatically on the rise in low- and middle-income countries, particularly in urban settings" (WHO 2017).

Obesity itself is presented as a self-evident "thing" that you can throw a rope around, a non-communicable and chronic disease, a spreading threat to nations, populations, and economic growth. There is a clear and generally accepted pattern of explanation for obesity. Firstly, it is identified by bodily measurements—with techniques and tools such as the BMI and ideal waist measurement (Hacking 2007; McCullough and Hardin 2013; Yates-Doerr 2013). *Fat Fighters* presented an animation of Australia's increasing BMI from 1980 to 2009, emphasizing the extra weight for men and women as equivalent to 180 donuts, or an adult female koala. Clinicians and epidemiologists agree that the BMI is not an exact science, but for the purpose of classifying bodily states (and conforming to medical classifications), it remains a ubiquitous standard against which our bodies are mapped and judged. Originating in epidemiology in the 1960s (but was not so named until 1972 by epidemiologist Ancel Keys (Hacking 2006, p. 88)), a BMI for adults aims to compare your weight to your height. Yates-Doerr (2013) notes that by the start of the twentieth century many US life insurance companies had used correlations of weight and height in their determinations of what constituted excessive fat (2013,

p. 53). While the parameters for what defined obesity remained somewhat fluid, the discursive fixing of certain body sizes (and their normal standards) came into play as an epidemiological tool. It wasn't until WHO and the National Institutes of Health standardized these terms in 1998 that the BMI became the pejorative classification of "underweight," a "healthy weight," "overweight," or "obese" for your height.

It is very easy and cheap to measure your BMI, and BMI calculators abound (Rich 2018). Such a simple number, however, carries significant meaning, and is used in US and UK school-based BMI measurement programs,[2] and even as an incentive for health insurance. Australia's national airline, Qantas, for example, provides an app to reward you for exercise, as well as a discount on life insurance premiums if you sit within the Heart Foundation's healthy BMI range.

With the discursive construction of universal and standardized BMIs, and the subsequent categorization of the normal and the pathological (Canguilhem 1966/1978), it becomes easier to identify overweight and obesity as either a health risk factor or a disease. Notwithstanding the disagreements as to whether obesity should be defined as a disease, it is now officially classified as a disease under the WHO's International Classification of Diseases. In June 2013 the American Medical Association officially classified obesity as a disease (a BMI above 30) (Stoner and Cornwall 2014). Clinicians in Canada are calling for obesity to be conceptualized as a "chronic disease" like type 2 diabetes or hypertension (Sharma et al. 2018) in order to qualify for comprehensive medical intervention. Australia has not followed this route and has not defined obesity as a disease, cautious of the stigmatizing effects of medicalizing so many people (who may be obese *and* also healthy).

The idea that being obese is a risk to health is extremely well cemented in many government and community attitudes and perceptions (Farrell et al. 2016; Olds et al. 2013). The Australian Government's Department of Health states: "The rates of overweight and obesity amongst adults have doubled over the past two decades, with Australia now being ranked as one of the fattest developed nations … and adults and adolescents aged more than 18 years who have a BMI greater than 25 kg/m^2 are at risk of, or have, one or more overweight or obesity-related co-morbidities" (Department of Health 2009). The health problems and consequences of obesity are extensively listed as

> *including musculo-skeletal problems, cardiovascular disease, some cancers, sleep apnea, type 2 diabetes, and hypertension, to name a few. Many of these are often preventable through a healthy and active lifestyle. In particular, obesity is strongly linked to type 2 diabetes, identified as one of the six National Health Priority Areas. There are several new, large well-conducted studies that have shown a clear relationship between excessive body weight and increased mortality and morbidity. Mortality and morbidity are also associated with the amount of weight gained in adult life. For example, a weight gain of 10 kg or more since young adulthood is associated with increased mortality, coronary heart disease, hypertension, stroke and type 2 diabetes.* (Australian Government 2009)

As expected in a neoliberal political climate, the economic consequences and costs of these chronic diseases are constructed as part of the problem. Obesity is identified not only as a major threat to health, but also to economic stability. The Australian Government suggests that the economic burden is "not only significant, but likely to get worse even if there is no further growth in the prevalence of obesity" (Australian Government 2009). International studies also sound this alarm bell, with "the World Economic Forum now ranking non-communicable diseases as one of the top global threats to economic development" (Bloom et al. 2011).

Beyond the critiques of the negative impacts of biopower through bodily measurement, there is an important caution with epidemiological evidence and its presentation. Despite the rhetoric concerning the rising tide of "globesity," Australian research has found that childhood weight increased between 1985 and 1996 but has not increased since 1997 (Booth et al. 2003; Hardy et al. 2012; Olds et al. 2010). In an analysis of 41 studies of childhood weight status in Australia, Olds et al. (2010) found that there was a "plateau in the percentage of boys and girls classified as overweight or obese, and that the prevalence had settled at around 21%–25% for overweight and obesity together, and at 5%–6% for obesity alone" (Olds et al. 2010, p. 57). Olds et al. (2011) also found that this plateauing effect could be observed in international trends in data from nine countries (including Australia, China, England, France, Netherlands, New Zealand, Sweden, Switzerland, and the USA). This could be explained by a number of hypotheses: an effect of interventions; we may have reached a point of saturation; that any child who is predisposed to overweight has become overweight; or that a sampling bias (due to stigmatization of obesity) has led to more parents declining to consent to their children being measured. Any or all of these factors could be at play, but as Olds et al. (2015) suggest, "[i]t's not yet time to uncork the Dom Perignon!" (2015, p. 22). One quarter of Australian children are overweight or obese and most do not meet the Australian physical activity guidelines.

There is also another important caveat to consider—that of social class. The relationship between social class and obesity is complex, and in developed countries there is strong evidence to demonstrate the inverse associations between socioeconomic indicators and obesity in adulthood (Offer et al. 2012; Ulijaszek 2012). While epidemiological evidence points to a flattening (or at the most to a "very small increase" (Olds et al. 2017, p. 481)) in the prevalence of obesity across Australia, certain sections of the population are identified as being more at risk of becoming obese. In Australia, as in most other developed nations, research suggests that obesity is more prevalent among families living in socioeconomic disadvantage (Ball and Crawford 2005; Hillier-Brown et al. 2014; MacFarlane et al. 2010; Peeters and Backholer 2014). A meta-analysis conducted by Olds et al. (2017) confirms that prevalence (and prevalence trends) varies across Australian states and territories. Upward prevalence trends appear in those states that are experiencing or have experienced significant economic challenges: Western Australia, South Australia, and Tasmania. For people experiencing disadvantage, socioeconomic inequalities are associated with poorer dietary intake, lower physical activity levels, and higher risks of obesity and cardiovascular diseases (Ball and Crawford 2005). Large bodies were visibly evident at our field site, with age-standardized rates of adult obesity twice as high in Playford (35.2%) than in more affluent suburbs of Adelaide (17.6%) (Australian Bureau of Statistics (ABS) 2014a; PHIDU 2014).

Obesity and social class are tied in what Ulijaszek (2012) calls "a transgenerational vicious circle," in that obesity can lead to low socioeconomic status and low socioeconomic status can lead to obesity. Studies in Europe have provided strong evidence to suggest that children who grow up in low socioeconomic households that are constrained by poor physical and social environments are more likely to develop obesity that persists into adulthood (Gnavi et al. 2001; Wardle et al. 2006).[3] Obesity is also socially stigmatized (Puhl and Latner 2007), and obese children "usually face social disadvantages in education, health care, and interpersonal relationships, as well as facing discrimination in employment when they become adults" (Ulijaszek 2012, p. 3).

As well as class, gender is also an important intersectional axis when looking at obesity prevalence. Recent evidence from the British National Child Development Study (1958–2008) confirms this trajectory associating children's obesity with future low socioeconomic status, but notes the higher penalty that women incur throughout their life course. Drawing on this birth cohort, Black et al. (2018) found that obesity at age 16 was associated with significantly lower levels of future household income for women, but not for men. In their analysis of 2011 data from the International Obesity Task Force, Wells et al. found that obesity among women is more common than obesity among men in almost all the populations they studied (74 countries). Interestingly, it was the countries that had greater gender equity where obesity was less prevalent (like Scandinavia) (Wells et al. 2012).

Gender differences are apparent in the Australian population, with women from lower socioeconomic circumstances and men from the middle classes having the highest rates of overweight and obesity (ABS 2013; Farrell et al. 2016). As food and eating is often central to women's roles in families, gender has obvious influences in how the debate unfolds, especially in the blaming of women for lack of good food provisioning in the family home due to "too many hours spent in the office" (Maher et al. 2010). Australian women living in low socioeconomic households are less likely to be able to afford healthy foods due to food insecurity (Foley et al. 2010) and have a range of competing priorities that make focusing on their well-being difficult. An earlier study we undertook in the same fieldwork location found that attention to achieving an idealized, thin, feminine body was not a priority, and was seen as a goal that middle-class women invest in (Warin et al. 2008). Desires for certain body shapes are, however, not just a gendered concern, but also intersect with race and class.

In her book on the geography of health inequalities, Clare Bambra suggests that "the relationship between socioeconomic status (SES) and health would not be assumed to be unidirectional and linear across the social gradient, but to function through multiple pathways operating at several different levels" (Bambra 2016, p. 109). This is perhaps most strikingly demonstrated in a recent UK study by Hughes and Kumari that examined associations of unemployment and BMI in a large, nationally representative study of UK adults (2017). This study found that the association between weight and employment was more of a U-shaped association, in that unemployed men from lower-income households tended to be very thin, but unemployed non-smoking men and women tended to be overweight. What this study reminds us is that the assumed direct pathway between obesity and low SES is non-linear and needs to be contextualized in relation to a range of modifying factors, such as age, gender roles, length of unemployment, smoking (which acts as an appetite suppressant), attitudes to and capacity for physical activity, social supports, mental illness or disability, and many other factors mechanistically linked to adiposity (Hughes and Kumari 2017). Socioeconomic status should thus "not be conceptualized as a basic cause exercising itself through specific mechanisms, but as an emergent property arising from patterned networked of social interaction" (Bambra 2016, p. 109).

When obesity is aggregated with gender and race, international studies point to obesity being more prevalent in racial/ethnic populations, with African-American women in the USA much more likely to be obese than the general population (Ogden et al. 2012). Similarly, in Australia, Indigenous Australians have high rates of obesity. The prevalence of overweight among young Aboriginal and Torres Strait Islander women (18–24 years) is almost double that of their non-Aboriginal peers (59% and 31% respectively) (ABS 2014b). Migrant groups are also disproportionately burdened by obesity and obesity-related disorders, but this differs according to length of time in Australia, and other sociocultural factors around food and gender (Renzaho et al. 2018).

There are clearly many ways in which obesity manifests between men and women of different cultural and ethnic backgrounds, including socioeconomic status. In interpreting all or any of the above metrics, we should remain cautious about "common-sense claims" that simply conflate fatness with disadvantage. We should also be circumspect, as many measurements of obesity are based on norms derived from white bodies (Guthman 2013b) and "remove situational context, leaving in its place abstract standards, quantitatively driven rules, and a focus on universal norms" (Yates-Doerr 2015, p. 163). Such "metrification" (ibid.) does not account for differing, or what Margaret Lock calls "local biologies" (Lock 1993). Local biologies understands bodies to be situationally placed, acknowledging the ways in which material bodies and their social environments interact to mediate experiences and symptoms. This concept highlights the need to understand *the contexts* of the social gradient, of how, for example, the discordant pleasure of foods helps to "make the bitter sweet" (Bissell et al. 2016; Zivkovic et al. 2015) and display resistance to middle-class perspectives on how bodies should behave.

Interestingly, Luke, one young male participant, captured this concept of local biologies when we asked him why the OPAL program was in his neighborhood:

> *The number of obese people you see in this area is probably, you see them, definitely. I think it is a significantly higher proportion in comparison to some of the more affluent suburbs. That probably depends a lot again on social circles and so on. Here, if you're very stereotypical, hey look, you've worked in the factory, the boys go down to the pub have a drink afterwards, go home have a meal and then sit in front of the TV. Very stereotypical. If you talk about an affluent suburb, one they are not in a factory; two they are in an office environment and go play squash after work. Completely different. They could be exactly the same physical person but five years down the track they've got very different profiles.*

Here, Luke acknowledges the ways in which one's *habitus* has an overwhelming impact on one's biology. The bodies of these men are embedded in and changed by their *habitus*—by their work circumstances (factories or offices), leisure preferences (a beer in the pub or playing squash), and the classed and gendered practices of everyday lives. The very different profiles Luke points to in terms of weight result from the "continuous exchange between the social and the biological in the production and reproduction of bodies in situated socio-cultural contexts" (Lock 2012).

Ulijaszek (2012) extends this argument, suggesting that all of these socioeconomic, gendered, and racially based factors are incomplete unless considered in the context of cultural capital. Drawing on Bourdieu's (1984) concept of symbolic capital, Ulijaszek argues that differing forms of capital (economic, social, and cultural) are utilized by different groups in society to amplify social stratification. Different values afforded to different foods and body sizes can be used to increase cultural capital; for example, African-American women perceive themselves to be healthier and more attractive to the opposite sex than white women of similar weight and age (Ulijaszek 2012). Preferences for body shapes and certain types of foods are factors that can lend prestige to certain groups, thus bolstering status. A common complaint we heard when talking to people about our research was along these lines: that people living in poverty say they can't afford healthy food, but they "all seem to have huge flat-screen televisions." In line with Ulijaszek's argument, we would argue that the capacity to participate in conspicuous consumption and purchase status technologies (and fast food) "endows status when in a broader societal context little else is available by which to mark status or symbolic capital" (Ulijaszek 2012, p. 5; c.f. Ulijaszek 2017, p. 85).

Dealing with a Wicked Problem

As many scholars have already noted (Coveney 2006; Gard and Wright 2005; Mayes 2016; Wright and Harwood 2009), obesity and its discontents is classic Foucauldian territory whereby you name a problem, use surveillance techniques to map it, and create a discourse using certain types of language and evidence (in this case, of epidemiological data, biostatistics, economic modeling, and disease classifications) to neatly circumscribe and hold this logic together. Once your problem is identified, solutions need to be developed to address the problem. Governments and a range of organizations step in to assemble the necessary apparatuses—an assembly of strategies, tactics, and procedures which inform and enact programs that target both populations and individuals (Coveney 2006, p. 146).

In 2013 the UN General Assembly described obesity as a "wicked problem." As a wicked problem obesity is said to be "highly resistant to resolution—not least because it's a moving target: everyone has different views on it (Ulijaszek 2017), and every attempt to fix it has consequences that complicate things further. There's no right way to solve a wicked problem" (Groves 2008). John Law (2014) digs further, arguing that wicked problems "are vicious, tricky, and aggressive, filled with political and material ambivalences, uncertainties and unpredictable feedback loops" (2014, p. 3). People search for ways to tame wicked problems, often in a managerial manner, on the presumption that things can be tamed by bringing everything together. This taming of an intractable problem was beautifully demonstrated by the crowded UK's Foresight Obesity Systems map, which we discuss in Chap. 4.

Obesity is not only a wicked problem but is also described as a "wicked policy problem," a "test case for 21st-century health policy" (Kickbusch and Buckett 2010, p. 13). As one might expect with public health responses, initiatives have favored education-based interventions (Lachat et al. 2013) rather than regulatory interventions. Responses to obesity in Australia have been mainly channeled through public education, social marketing, and, to a lesser extent, community-wide initiatives that focus on changing diets and/or physical activity. Because obesity is broadly perceived as an individual problem related to poor choices (Farrell et al. 2015, 2016; Thibodeau and Flusberg 2017), these strategies win public support (Swinburn et al. 2011, p. 810) and aim to provide relevant information in order to encourage and "nudge" people to change their behaviors and adopt a healthier lifestyle.

In the last two decades in Australia there have been many obesity-related interventions delivered at national, state, and local levels. Initiatives include making people aware of nutrition guidelines and physical activity: for example, the *Go for 2 & 5* national campaign; *Smart Choices*, a mandatory Queensland Government strategy; a national training manual developed through *Eat Smart, Play Smart* for out-of-school hours care, reducing screen time in family homes, educating people about the link between increased waist measurement and the risk of chronic disease, such as heart disease and type 2 diabetes (*Measure Up* campaign); how to swap unhealthy foods for more healthy foods (*Swap It. Don't Stop It*); and the *Eat Well Be Active* community-based program in South Australia. No longer an uncommon affliction and sleepy academic topic, obesity has been elevated to high political status. It was on this accelerating train of obesity health interventions that OPAL arrived in South Australia—grander in scale and more ambitious in scope.

A Counter Discourse: More "Obesity Wars"

The metaphorical rendering of obesity as an "epidemic" and a "time bomb," and those who are obese as a "threat," generates a language of panic and fear (Evans 2010; Monaghan et al. 2013). An OPAL manager agreed: "The prevalence of obesity is obviously scary." Obesity is described as "an impending economic and social catastrophe" (Neel 2011) and "a deadly health crisis" (Neel 2011), and these metaphors have implications for how we come to understand obesity and treat people who are obese. Bombak argues that science is used to rationalize this fear: "Individuals should fear fat because science assures us that fat threatens the health of individuals and nations and is reflective of individuals' modern behavioral weaknesses" (Bombak 2014, p. 517). The language of fear and risk immediately implies danger, and danger, in turn, implies harm.

Not everyone agrees with these dire characterizations of fat, and a significant body of work has developed to counter the medicalization of obesity and popular representations. The women from *Fat Fighters* described at the beginning of this chapter represent one outpost of this group, clearly rallying against the stigmatization and medicalization of fatness and calling for an end to "fat shaming." In the academic and activist world, critical fat scholars work to leverage Foucault's incisive critique of biopower and deviant bodies, taking issue with the pervasive cultural movement of "fat phobia."

The field of fat and obesity studies is not homogeneous. As scholars have well described, there is a diverse range of critical perspectives on the dominant positioning of obesity that offer both complementary and conflicting viewpoints (for overviews, see Wright and Harwood 2009; Gard 2011; Warin 2014; Bombak 2014; Monaghan et al. 2010).

Critical fat scholars are well known for presenting early arguments that critiqued dominant biomedical explanations. Drawing on social constructionist frames, writers such as Campos (2004), Gard and Wright (2001, 2005), and Saguy and Riley (2005) downplayed the moral panic associated with the "obesity epidemic and crisis" in order to unpack the powerful tropes that this discourse relied upon. Some scholars went further, taking a "hard" (Guthman 2013b) social constructionist position to describe obesity science as a "state science" (Holmes et al. 2006) in which "the fabrication of evidence in obesity research constitutes a good example of micro-fascism at play in the contemporary scientific arena" (Rail et al. 2010, p. 259; c.f. Davis et al. 2008).

Another group of activists and scholars took a slightly different post-structuralist angle, and questioned the direct link made between ill-health and weight. The fat acceptance, fat activism, and Health at Every Size (HAES) movements rallied against the social injustices that accompany weight stigmatization and emphasized diversity through "size acceptance, fat acceptance, fat liberation and fat politics" (Cooper 1998, 2009, 2010). The passion to change sociocultural perceptions of obesity led to a collective call to arms, perhaps exemplified by Rothblum and Solovay (2009) in their edited book *Fat Studies Reader*, where readers are incited to join the "revolution" against the medicalization of fatness.

Many of these critiques have proved to be indispensable to understanding the medicalization (and biomedicalization) of bodies, the moral panic of the "obesity epidemic," the limits of the body mass index (BMI) as a universal metric (Evans and Colls 2009; Oliver 2006; Ross 2005), the direct association between obesity and ill-health (Aphramor 2005; Aphramor et al. 2013) and subsequent pathologization of fat (Gard and Wright 2005), neoliberal forms of obesity governance (Wright and Harwood 2009), reductionist and decontextualized accounts of obesity, and the demonization of particular groups of people who are more "at risk" of obesity (children, disadvantaged populations across race and class, and mothers) (Warin et al. 2008, 2012; Zivkovic et al. 2010; Boero 2007; Richardson 2015).

Unsurprisingly, this scholarship can be challenging for those coming from a more biomedical or clinical perspective. Reviewing a recent book entitled *Obesity in Canada* (2016), edited by three well-known critical fat scholars, Sharma (a professor of medicine and chair in obesity research) sums up the overall position from critical fat studies scholars in this edition:

> *There is no global obesity epidemic, the health consequences of obesity are over-blown, and measures aimed at preventing or treating obesity are a thinly-veiled conspiracy by the biomedical establishment to create a moral panic that justifies the reassertion of normative identities pertaining to gender, race, class, and sexuality.* (Sharma 2017, p. 499)

In this intensely political space of contestation, there are disagreements within fields, as the study of Flegal and colleagues demonstrates. Their systematic review shocked obesity scientists when they found that "obesity overall was not associated with higher mortality, and overweight was associated with significantly lower all-cause mortality" (Flegal et al. 2013). The study was quickly derided by many in the clinical realm as "a pile of rubbish … and no-one should waste their time reading it" (Aubrey 2013, cited in Bombak 2014, p. 517). Of course, critical fat scholars were delighted with this news, and used the authoritative power of scientific evidence to their advantage.

These disparate and conflicting discourses illustrate the power struggles for legitimacy and authority in the obesity space. These conflicts exemplify the definition of a field given by Bourdieu and Wacquant as

> *a network, or a configuration, of objective relations between positions. These positions are objectively defined, in their existence and in the determinations they impose upon their occupants, agents or institutions, by their present and potential situation … in the structure of the distribution of species of power (or capital) whose possession commands access to the specific profits that are at stake in the field, as well as be their objective relation to other positions (domination, subordination, homology).* (Bourdieu and Wacquant 1992, p. 97)

In other words, there are multiple agents and institutions vying for the loudest and most legitimate voice in determining what obesity is and how the problem is diagnosed and dealt with. Social scientists will have different epistemological training from clinicians, and each field will come armed with a store of knowledge that underpins the ways in which they see obesity. And of course, within social sciences and clinical fields there will be many fields, each struggling to position itself in an array of competing and conflicting knowledges. There are hierarchies of disciplinary knowledge within universities and funding bodies, and from a position of power they operate to elevate and maintain some forms of knowledge at the expense of others or against multiple ways of knowing (c.f. Kenney and Müller 2018). In obesity studies, the medical field has the most power through its discursive acquisition of symbolic authority, and all other fields struggle to gain legitimacy.

Trapped in the Problem

In acknowledging the interplay of fields and the positioning of differing hierarchies of knowledge, we argue that the problem we were investigating was already (and ironically) closed even before our research began. Guthman's concept of problem closure provides a helpful view of the circumscribed space in which we were caught:

> *[It is a] situation when a specific definition of a problem is used to frame subsequent study of the problem's causes and consequences in ways that preclude alternative conceptualizations of the problem* (Hajer 1995, p. 22) … *it may entail embedding assumptions about a scientific object's character into the research of that object* (Jasanoff 2004; Reardon 2005) … *or defining the cause of the problem in relation to socially acceptable solutions* (Forsyth 2003). (Guthman 2013a, p. 143)

We were complicit in this process as our grant proposal, which funded this research, used the "problem of obesity" as leverage to investigate whether families in our proposed fieldwork site conceptualized obesity in terms of risk. Our study aimed to work in with Australia's largest childhood obesity program and had significant financial backing from three tiers of government. All the promotional material and rationale for the OPAL program took the "problem" of obesity for granted. The South Australian Government supported OPAL as they were "committed to tackling the serious public health concern of overweight and obesity" in the state. OPAL marketing drew upon discourses of "acting now" (Evans 2010; Warin et al. 2015), stating that "experts have warned that unless the obesity problem is addressed, the current generation of children could die younger than their parents" (OPAL State Coordination Unit 2009). The OPAL Scientific Advisory Committee (comprising academic experts mainly from health sciences) was formed to support the initiative and ensure evidence-based approaches directed it.

Our grant was notionally an industry collaboration and, as we detail in the next chapter, we worked closely with state government and non-governmental organizations (NGOs), and the local council of the area where our research was to be carried out. At the time, obesity had been designated as a national priority by the Australian Government, and the OPAL program was clearly addressing this priority. It is important to be clear that as a research team we did not hold strong social constructionist views about obesity. While critical of the biopolitics of obesity discourses, we did not view obesity as a fabricated issue. We *did* recognize problems around obesity: for example, the health inequities that underpin its prevalence, and the need to understand how people in the community experienced and understood their "risky bodies." Moreover, we would never have secured external funding partners had we presented a counter discourse to dominant obesity models, as the grant expected alignment in how the problem was understood and presented, and how we could work together to address it. This crucially raises the question of how university researchers can partner with external bodies or whether funding schemes are complicit in upholding dominant discourses.

In all of our preliminary meetings to discuss the grant proposal, there were nods in agreement about the "problem of obesity," and how an anthropological project could explore concepts of risk and resistance to obesity interventions. At one meeting with a local councilor at the fieldwork site, we were told that as long as we didn't "ride in on our white horses" our project would be approved. This community has long been a site for intervention and research, with a raft of well-intentioned professionals (do-gooders) coming to save people from their seemingly dire circumstances.

Defining obesity to begin with as a negative problem of risk that must be prevented or slowed is a classic example of problem closure (Guthman 2013a, p. 144). This narrowing of the problem definition has been described thus: "These spaces collectively enact a problem space around obesity, and they outline the contours of possible interventions" (Sanabria 2016, p. 142). Any alternative understanding or resistance to the received "truths" of obesity were outside this space and therefore difficult to voice.

Our external partners' explanations for the relationship between obesity and disadvantage were premised on a lack of access to and education about nutritious foods, the ubiquity and affordability of unhealthy food, and a dearth of appropriate recreational spaces. In her own work on obesity, Guthman (2013a) suggests that such assumptions about what impels behaviors in "obesogenic" areas operate to foreclose alternative conceptualizations of the relationship between obesity and socioeconomic disadvantage. Hence, any of our findings that demonstrated resistance to healthy eating, unwillingness to eat a healthy breakfast, or, conversely, gave positive accounts of large bodies were immediately negated and/or dismissed.

The dominant construction of obesity means that the problem is always deflected back to individuals, who are seen to have specific deficiencies and to lack knowledge about what to eat, how to eat, or how to treat their bodies. In ethnographic observations from policy spaces, scientific forums, and international advocacy groups, describing how knowledge circulates in "obesity epidemic" discourses, Sanabria (2016) brings the "play of ignorance" into perspective. In line with much of the recent literature on knowing/not-knowing, she argues that the prevailing consensus about the problem of obesity operates as a politics of ignorance.

We are not suggesting that participants in our field site were ignorant, or that any of our external partners were, or the OPAL staff. The circulation of ignorance is much more implicit. The current idea that people simply need to be educated about health through health promotion information and social marketing "nudges" is based on an outdated model of hierarchical knowledge in which people are constructed as empty vessels waiting to be filled up with the "right knowledge." Once equipped with new knowledge, such as how much sugar is in soft drinks, or that some cereals contain more fiber and "goodness" than others, people are expected to change their behaviors accordingly. Sanabria says that while this model is "quaint" (Sanabria 2016, p. 137), and despite evidence that this transfer of knowledge does not work, this type of health education remains entrenched and continues to be promoted among experts (ibid., p. 137).

To anthropologists it should come as no surprise that there were discrepancies in how our external partners and community members thought about obesity. There were numerous perspectives on obesity and nutrition and these types of differences have been well documented in other ethnographies and critical dietetics (Warin et al. 2008; Yates-Doerr 2012, 2015; Biltekoff et al. 2014; Scrinis 2013). But there are problems with leaving the analysis here. In pointing to the different Bourdieurian fields of knowledge that circulate around obesity (from nutritionists, community workers, community members, social marketers, anthropologists, and local government), each explanation is hermetically sealed in its own epistemological bubble. Lay knowledge and expert knowledge are compared, and ethnographic authority rests with the former. In the field, however, these spaces were not sealed, and leaked into one another.

Perspectival Tales

Sometime before Guthman's discussion of problem closure, Mol (2002) was warning about the dangers of such perspectival tales in her book *The Body Multiple*. She describes what happens when the problem—in our case obesity—is placed "in the middle of a circle [and a] crowd of silent faces assembles around it. They seem to get to know the object by their eyes only" (Mol 2002, p. 12). People will have different perspectives on what the thing is, and how it is constructed, made meaningful, and experienced. The problem with this type of analysis is that it leaves the physical reality of the body untouched, and we are trapped in disease categories that naturalize large bodies as negative. It's as if the category of obesity is a "reality out there for everyone to stumble over before interpreting it in diverse ways … people's categories … do not reflect a nature accessible … instead, they are part of a specific practice for dealing with life, suffering and death" (Mol 2002, p. 24).

As the title of Mol's book attests, the body is multiple. Rather than fix the object of inquiry as a central focus, Mol suggests that ethnographers might look toward events in practice, the relationships between events, and the embedded knowledges entailed in them. This includes some of the ethnographic data we could not speak or write about to our industry partners during our fieldwork. When the food bank volunteers from the local community were told to change the food items on their shelves to healthier options, and only promote what they referred to as "boring food," they carefully negotiated the circulation of "something nice" for local shoppers. Chocolates were cautiously bought and sold. At times they would alert each other with excited whispers when council workers eager to "reshape" Playford were about to enter the store, and with rushed hands hid all the contraband chocolates and biscuits under the counter. On other occasions, salty ingredients (such as packaged parmesan cheese) were snuck into healthy OPAL recipes that were made on site and offered to customers to entice them to change their cooking tastes and behaviors. There were many small acts of resistance to the perceived policing of daily pleasures. We quickly realized that participants were telling us things that they were not telling OPAL staff and that practices around eating were constantly manipulated in their everyday worlds. Some felt that the black and white rules of healthy eating were "taking away food choices"—at times they were pretending to go along with OPAL but once out of sight and earshot they made jokes and criticized the program. One participant recognized the ways in which she slid between different performances: "I'm actually living in two worlds—I'm living in the local government world and the reality world which is here [in this community]." Tactics of *la perruque* were clearly in operation: "Sly as a fox and twice as quick: there are countless ways of 'making do'" (de Certeau 1984, p. 29).

We could not report on some of this material at the time because it was imperative that we protected people's jobs and volunteering roles. This became a major problem in the research project, for we could not disclose these subversive practices and also maintain participant anonymity. OPAL staff were understandably very cautious about the program being perceived as a failure and made every attempt to avoid any negative media coverage. Our grant contract required us to give all written papers and presentations to each external partner for review prior to publication or public dissemination. At times we were asked to withdraw conference presentations or alter academic publications. Even brand names of products in academic publications (such as Kellogg's®) were asked to be removed as it was feared that large food industry corporations—that we were told searched for negative press releases—could take legal action. We found ourselves being risk-managed and were asked explicitly to provide "more palatable" versions of our findings for bureaucratic consumption.

In this chapter we have shown that obesity is not a single entity and that the facts of obesity are continually being contested. The body, as Mol argues (and as we saw from *The Fat Fighters* program), is multiple and there are various enactments of obesity. This is the point that Jeanette Pols makes in her assessment of Emily Yates-Doerr's (2015) ethnography of obesity in postwar Guatemala:

> *If obesity is not one thing that can be defined on a singular scale, you cannot say something general and coherent about it. Obesity is indeed a problem to the people in Xela, but it manifests itself in very different ways. So, we need to ask* ***how*** *it is a problem,* ***where*** *and* ***for whom****. We need to ask: what* ***is*** *obesity, in this particular practice? There is no general thing called obesity. There are only local practices in which obesity is shaped through the ways it is framed and handled. There are many different problems of obesity. As there are many kinds of health.* (Pols 2016)

It is important to place politics front and center in any study of obesity, especially in an ethnographic study. Obesity is rife with politics: the politics of who can speak about obesity; who holds authority; who has the best solution to address obesity; the politics of stigma; the politics of risk, class, gender, and race; and the politics of morality and lifestyles. Mol prefers to write about these types of politics as coexistences—of how different versions of a "single object" (here, obesity) coexist (2002, p. 180). These coexistences will never flatten out, and entail discord, tension, contrast, multiplicity, interdependence, distribution, inclusion, enactment, practice, and enquiry (2002, pp. 180–181). This is also our point of departure in this book. We are not interested in who is right and who is wrong, but interested in discerning the patterns of these relationships and in understanding how fatness and obesity are practiced.

Notes

1. For an excellent overview of the rationalities of differing models of obesity in the last 40 years, see Ulijaszek (2017).
2. In their analysis of the UK's National Child Measurement Programme (NCMP), Evans and Colls (2009) note the incidence of "heavier children" opting out of BMI monitoring. Despite this obvious effect of stigmatization and the limitations of the BMI as a measurement of health, Evans and Colls suggest that the continued measurement of children's height and weight and reporting back to parents is an exemplar of "governmental efficiency of shame" (Evans and Colls 2009, p. 1077).
3. Simmonds et al. (2016) conducted a systematic review to investigate if obese children and adolescents are likely to become obese adults. They found that when measured with BMI, adolescent obesity is likely to persist into adulthood. However, the study also found that most obese adults were not obese in childhood, and "targeting weight-reduction interventions specifically at obese or overweight children, although potentially beneficial for those children, is therefore unlikely to have a substantial impact on reducing the overall obesity burden in adulthood" (Simmonds et al. 2016, p. 103).

References

Aphramor, L. (2005). Is a weight-centred health framework salutogenic? Some thoughts on unhinging certain dietary ideologies. *Social Theory & Health, 3*(4), 315–340.

Aphramor, L., Brady, J., & Gingras, J. (2013). Advancing critical dietetics: Theorising health at every size. In E. Abbotts & A. Lavis (Eds.), *Why we eat, how we eat: Contemporary encounters between foods and bodies* (pp. 85–102). Farnham: Ashgate.

Aubrey, A. (2013). Research: A little extra fat may help you live longer. *Morning Edition*. Available: Health/168437030.

Australian Bureau of Statistics (ABS). (2013). Australian Health Survey: Updated Results, 2011–12 [Internet]. Catalogue no. 4364.0.55.003. Available at http://www.abs.gov.au/ausstats/abs@.nsf/Lookup/4364.0.55.003main+features12011-2012. Accessed 14 Nov 2017.

Australian Bureau of Statistics (ABS). (2014a). *Community profiles*. http://www.abs.gov.au/websitedbs/censushome.nsf/home/communityprofiles. Accessed 14 Nov 2017.

Australian Bureau of Statistics (ABS). (2014b). *Australian Aboriginal and Torres Strait Islander Health Survey: First Results*, 2012–13. http://www.abs.gov.au/ausstats/abs@.nsf/mf/4727.0.55.001. Accessed 14 Nov 2017.

Australian Government, Department of Health. (2009). *About overweight and obesity*. http://www.health.gov.au/internet/main/publishing.nsf/content/health-pubhlth-strateg-hlthwt-obesity.htm

Ball, K., & Crawford, D. (2005). Socioeconomic status and weight change in adults: A review. *Social Science & Medicine, 60*, 1987–2010.

Bambra, C. (2016). *Health divides: Where you live can kill you*. Bristol: Policy Press.

Berlant, L. (2011). *Cruel optimism*. London: Duke University Press.

Biltekoff, C., Mudry, J., Kimura, A. H., Landecker, H., & Guthman, J. (2014). Interrogating moral and quantification discourses in nutritional knowledge. *Gastronomica: The Journal of Critical Food Studies, 14*(3), 17–26.

Bissell, P., Peacock, M., Blackburn, J., & Smith, C. (2016). The discordant pleasures of everyday eating: Reflections on the social gradient in obesity under neo-liberalism. *Social Science & Medicine, 159*, 14–21.

Black, N., Kung, C. S., & Peeters, A. (2018). For richer, for poorer: The relationship between adolescent obesity and future household economic prosperity. *Preventive Medicine, 111*, 142–150.

Bloom, D. E., Cafiero, E. T., Jané-Llopis, E., et al. (2011). *The global economic burden of non-communicable diseases*. Geneva: World Economic Forum.

Boero, N. (2007). All the news that's fat to print: The American 'obesity epidemic' and the media. *Qualitative Sociology, 30*(1), 41–60.

Bombak, A. (2014). The 'obesity epidemic': Evolving science, unchanging etiology. *Sociology Compass, 8*(5), 509–524.

Booth, M. L., Chey, T., Wake, M., Norton, K., Hesketh, K., Dollman, J., & Robertson, I. (2003). Change in the prevalence of overweight and obesity among young Australians, 1969–1997. *The American Journal of Clinical Nutrition, 77*(1), 29–36.

Bourdieu, P. (1984). *Distinction: A social critique of the judgment of taste* (trans: Nice, R.). Cambridge: Harvard University Press.

Bourdieu, P., & Wacquant, L. J. (1992). *An invitation to reflexive sociology.* Chicago: University of Chicago Press.

Campos, P. (2004). *The obesity myth.* New York: Gotham Books.

Canguilhem, G. (1966/1978). *On the normal and the pathological.* Dordrecht: Reidel Publishing.

Cooper, C. (1998). *Fat and proud: The politics of size.* London: The Women's Press.

Cooper, C. (2009). Fat activism in ten astonishing, beguiling, inspiring and beautiful episodes. In C. Tomrley & N. A. Kaloski (Eds.), *Fat studies in the UK* (pp. 19–31). York: Raw Nerve Books.

Cooper, C. (2010). Fat studies: Mapping the field. *Sociology Compass, 4*(12), 1020–1034.

Coveney, J. (2006). *Food, morals and meaning: The pleasure and anxiety of eating* (2nd ed.). London: Routledge.

Davis, B., Rich, E., Evans, J., & Allwood, R. (2008). *Education, disordered eating and obesity discourse: Fat fabrications.* London: Routledge.

De Certeau, M. D. (1984). *The practice of everyday life.* Berkeley: University of California Press.

Evans, B. (2010). Anticipating fatness: Childhood, affect, and the pre-emptive war on obesity. *Transactions of the Institute of British Geographers, 35*, 21–38.

Evans, B., & Colls, R. (2009). Measuring fatness, governing bodies: The spatialities of the Body Mass Index (BMI) in anti-obesity politics. *Antipode, 41*(5), 1051–1083.

Farrell, L. C., Warin, M. J., Moore, V. M., & Street, J. M. (2015). Emotion in obesity discourse: Understanding public attitudes towards regulations for obesity prevention. *Sociology of Health and Illness, 38*(4), 554–558.

Farrell, L. C., Warin, M. J., Moore, V. M., & Street, J. M. (2016). Socio-economic divergence in public opinions about preventive obesity regulations: Is the purpose to 'make some things cheaper, more affordable' or to 'help them get over their own ignorance'? *Social Science and Medicine, 154*, 1–8.

Flegal, K. M., Kit, B. K., Orpana, H., & Graubard, B. I. (2013). Association of all-cause mortality with overweight and obesity using standard Body Mass Index categories: A systematic review and meta-analysis. *JAMA: The Journal of the American Medical Association, 309*(1), 71–82.

Foley, W., Ward, P., Carter, P., Coveney, J., Tsourtos, G., & Taylor, A. (2010). An ecological analysis of factors associated with food insecurity in South Australia, 2002–07. *Public Health Nutrition, 13*(2), 215–221.

Gard, M. (2011). Truth, belief and the cultural politics of obesity scholarship and public health policy. *Critical Public Health, 21*(1), 37–48.

Gard, M., & Wright, J. (2001). Managing uncertainty: Obesity discourses and physical education in a risk society. *Studies in Philosophy and Education, 20*(6), 535–549.

Gard, M., & Wright, J. (2005). *The obesity epidemic: Science, morality and ideology*. London: Routledge.

Gnavi, R., Spagnoli, T. D., Galotto, C., Pugliese, E., Carta, A., & Cesari, L. (2001). Socioeconomic status, overweight and obesity in prepubertal children: A study in an area of Northern Italy. *European Journal of Epidemiology, 16*, 797–803.

Groves, T. (2008). National obesity strategy: What's the big idea? *British Medical Journal, 337*. https://doi.org/10.1136/bmj.a2548.

Guthman, J. (2013a). Too much food and too little sidewalk? Problematizing the obesogenic environment thesis. *Environment and Planning, 45*(1), 142–158.

Guthman, J. (2013b). Fatuous measures: The artifactual construction of the obesity epidemic. *Critical Public Health, 23*(3), 263–273.

Hacking, I. (2006). Genetics, biosocial groups & the future of identity. *Daedalus, 135*(4), 81–95.

Hacking, I. (2007). Where did the BMI come from? In P. Jonvallen (Ed.), *Bodies of evidence: Fat across disciplines*. Cambridge: Cambridge University.

Hajer, M. A. (1995). *The politics of environmental discourse: Ecological modernization and the policy process*. New York: Oxford University Press.

Hardy, L. L., Cosgrove, C., King, L., Venugopal, K., Baur, L. A., & Gill, T. (2012). Shifting curves? Trends in thinness and obesity among Australian youth, 1985 to 2010. *Pediatric Obesity, 7*(2), 92–100.

Hillier-Brown, F. C., Bambra, C. L., Cairns, J. M., Kasim, A., Moore, H. J., & Summerbell, C. D. (2014). A systematic review of the effectiveness of individual, community and societal level interventions at reducing socioeconomic inequalities in obesity amongst children. *BMC Public Health, 14*(1), 834.

Holmes, D., Murray, S., Perron, A., & Rail, G. (2006). Deconstructing the evidence-based discourse in health sciences: Truth, power, and fascism. *International Journal of Evidence-Based Healthcare, 4*(3), 180–186.

Hughes, A., & Kumari, M. (2017). Unemployment, underweight, and obesity: Findings from Understanding Society (UKHLS). *Preventive Medicine, 97*, 19–25.

Jasanoff, S. (2004). *States of knowledge: The co-production of science and social order*. London: Routledge.

Kenney, M., & Müller, R. (2018). Of rats and women: Narratives of motherhood in environmental epigenetics. In *The Palgrave handbook of biology and society* (pp. 799–830). London: Palgrave Macmillan.

Kickbusch, I., & Buckett, K. (2010). *Implementing health in all policies: Adelaide 2010* (pp. 11–24). Adelaide: Health in All Policies Unit, SA Department of Health.

Lachat, C., Otchere, S., Roberfroid, D., Abdulai, A., Seret, F., Milesevic, J., Kolsteren, P., et al. (2013). Diet and physical activity for the prevention of noncommunicable diseases in low-and middle-income countries: A systematic policy review. *PLoS Medicine, 10*(6), e1001465.

Law, J. (2014). *Working well with wickedness.* CRESC (Centre for Research on Socio-Cultural Change) working paper. Retrieved from http://www.cresc.ac.uk/publications/working-well-with-wickedness

Lock, M. (1993). *Encounters with aging: Mythologies of menopause in Japan and North America.* Berkeley: University of California Press.

Lock, M. (2012). The epigenome and nature/nurture reunification: A challenge for anthropology. *Medical Anthropology, 32*(4), 291–308.

MacFarlane, A., Abbott, G., Crawford, D., & Ball, K. (2010). Personal, social and environmental correlates of healthy weight status amongst mothers from socio-economically disadvantaged neighborhoods: Findings from the READI study. *International Journal of Behavioral Nutrition and Physical Activity, 7*(1), 23.

Maher, J., Fraser, S., & Wright, J. (2010). Framing the mother: Childhood obesity, maternal responsibility and care. *Journal of Gender Studies, 19*(3), 233–247.

Mayes, C. (2016). *The biopolitics of lifestyle: Foucault, ethics and healthy choices.* New York: Routledge.

McCullough, M. B., & Hardin, J. A. (Eds.). (2013). *Reconstructing obesity: The meaning of measures and the measure of meanings* (Vol. 2). New York: Berghahn Books.

Mol, A. (2002). *The body multiple: Ontology in medical practice.* Durham: Duke University Press.

Monaghan, L., Hollands, R., & Pritchard, G. (2010). Obesity epidemic entrepreneurs: Types, practices and interests. *Body & Society, 16*(2), 37–71.

Monaghan, L., Colls, R., & Evans, B. (Eds.). (2013). *Obesity discourse and fat politics: Research, critique and interventions.* London: Routledge.

NCD Risk Factor Collaboration. (2016). Trends in adult body-mass index in 200 countries from 1975 to 2014: A pooled analysis of 1698 population-based measurement studies with 19.2 million participants. *The Lancet, 387*(10026), 1377–1396.

Neel, D. (2011). *A wicked problem: Combating obesity in the developing world.* Harvard College Global Health Review. Retrieved from https://www.hcs.harvard.edu/hghr/online/obesity-developing/

Offer, A., Pechey, R., & Ulijaszek, S. (2012). *Insecurity, inequality, and obesity in affluent societies.* Oxford: Oxford University Press.

Ogden, C. L., Carroll, M. D., Kit, B. K., & Flegal, K. M. (2012). Prevalence of obesity in the United States, 2009–2010. *NCHS Data Brief, 82*, 1e8.

Olds, T. S., Tomkinson, G. R., Ferrar, K. E., & Maher, C. A. (2010). Trends in the prevalence of childhood overweight and obesity in Australia between 1985 and 2008. *International Journal of Obesity, 34*(1), 57–66.

Olds, T. I. M., Maher, C., Zumin, S. H. I., Péneau, S., Lioret, S., Castetbon, K., & Lissner, L. (2011). Evidence that the prevalence of childhood overweight is plateauing: Data from nine countries. *International Journal of Pediatric Obesity, 6*(5–6), 342–360.

Olds, T., Thomas, S., Lewis, S., & Petkov, J. (2013). Clustering of attitudes towards obesity: A mixed methods study of Australian parents and children. *International Journal of Behavioral Nutrition and Physical Activity, 10*(1), 117.

Olds, T., Schranz, N., & Tomkinson, G. (2015). Have we reached peak fat? *Sport Health, 33*, 20–22. https://sma.org.au/sma-site-content/uploads/2017/08/Sport-Health-Issue-1-2015.pdf

Olds, T., Schranz, N., & Maher, C. (2017). Secular trends in the prevalence of childhood overweight and obesity across Australian states: A meta-analysis. *Journal of Science and Medicine in Sport, 20*(5), 480–488.

Oliver, E. (2006). *Fat politics: The real story behind America's obesity epidemic*. Oxford: Oxford University Press.

OPAL State Coordination Unit. (2009). *OPAL (obesity prevention and lifestyle)*. Adelaide: Department of Health, Government of South Australia.

Peeters, A., & Backholer, K. (2014). Prioritising and tackling socio-economic inequalities in obesity. *BMC Obesity, 1*(1), 16.

Pols, J. (2016, November 13). Response to 'The Weight of Obesity'. *Somatosphere*. http://somatosphere.net/forumpost/response-to-the-weight-of-obesity-4

Public Health Information Development Unit (PHIDU). (2014). *Social health atlas of Australia*. Public Health Information Development Unit, University of Adelaide. http://www.adelaide.edu.au/phidu/help-info/about-our-data/indicators-notes/sha-aust/

Puhl, R. M., & Latner, J. D. (2007). Stigma, obesity, and the health of the nation's children. *Psychology Bulletin, 133*, 557–580.

Rail, G., Holmes, D., & Murray, S. J. (2010). The politics of evidence on 'domestic terrorists': Obesity discourses and their effects. *Social Theory & Health, 8*(3), 259–279.

Reardon, J. (2005). *Race to the finish: Identity and governance in an age of genomics*. Princeton: Princeton University Press.

Renzaho, A. M., Green, J., Smith, B. J., & Polonsky, M. (2018). Exploring factors influencing childhood obesity prevention among migrant communities in Victoria, Australia: A qualitative study. *Journal of Immigrant and Minority Health, 20*(4), 865–883.

Rich, E. (2018). Healthism, girls' embodiment, and contemporary health and physical education: From weight management to digital practices of optimization. In *The Palgrave handbook of feminism and sport, leisure and physical education* (pp. 523–536). London: Palgrave Macmillan.

Richardson, S. (2015). Maternal bodies in the postgenomic order: Gender and the explanatory landscape of epigenetics. In S. Richardson (Ed.), *Postgenomics*. Durham: Duke University Press.

Ross, B. (2005). Fat or fiction: Weighing the obesity epidemic. In M. Gard & J. Wright (Eds.), *The obesity epidemic: Science, morality and ideology*. London: Routledge.

Rothblum, E. D., & Solovay, S. (Eds.). (2009). *The fat studies reader*. New York: New York University Press.

Saguy, A., & Riley, K. (2005). Weighing both sides: Morality, mortality, and framing contests over obesity. *Journal of Health Politics, Policy and Law, 30*, 869–923.

Sanabria, E. (2016). Circulating ignorance: Complexity and agnogenesis in the obesity 'epidemic'. *Cultural Anthropology, 31*(1), 131–158.

Scrinis, G. (2013). *Nutritionism: The science and politics of dietary advice*. New York: Columbia University Press.

Sharma, A. (2017). Critical fat studies and obesity in Canada. *The Lancet, Diabetes and Endocrinology, 5*(7), 499–500.

Sharma, A. M., Goodwin, D. L., & Causgrove Dunn, J. (2018). Conceptualizing obesity as a chronic disease: An interview with Dr. Arya Sharma. *Adapted Physical Activity Quarterly, 20*, 1–8.

Simmonds, M., Llewellyn, A., Owen, C. G., & Woolacott, N. (2016). Predicting adult obesity from childhood obesity: A systematic review and meta-analysis. *Obesity Reviews, 17*(2), 95–107.

Stoner, L., & Cornwall, J. (2014). Did the American Medical Association make the correct decision classifying obesity as a disease? *The Australasian Medical Journal, 7*(11), 462.

Swinburn, B. A., Sacks, G., Hall, K. D., McPherson, K., Finegood, D. T., Moodie, M. L., & Gortmaker, S. L. (2011). The global obesity pandemic: Shaped by global drivers and local environments. *The Lancet, 378*(9793), 804–814.

Thibodeau, P. H., & Flusberg, S. J. (2017). Lay theories of obesity: Causes and consequences. In J. Gordeladze (Ed.). *Adiposity: Epidemiology and treatment modalities*. London: IntechOpen. https://www.intechopen.com/books/adiposity-epidemiology-and-treatment-modalities/lay-theories-of-obesity-causes-and-consequences

Ulijaszek, S. J. (2012). Socio-economic status, forms of capital and obesity. *Journal of Gastrointestinal Cancer, 43*(1), 3–7.

Ulijaszek, S. J. (2017). *Models of obesity: From ecology to complexity in science and policy*. Cambridge: Cambridge University Press.

Wardle, J., Brodersen, N. H., Cole, T. J., Jarvis, M. J., & Boniface, D. R. (2006). Development of adiposity in adolescence: Five-year longitudinal study of an ethnically and socioeconomically diverse sample of young people in Britain. *British Medical Journal, 332*(7550), 1130–1135.

Warin, M. (2014). Material feminism, obesity science and the limits of discursive critique. *Body & Society, 21*(4), 48–76.

Warin, M., Turner, K., Moore, V., & Davies, M. (2008). Bodies, mothers and identities: Rethinking obesity and the BMI. *Sociology of Health & Illness, 30*(1), 97–111.

Warin, M., Zivkovic, T., Davies, M., & Moore, V. (2012). Mothers as smoking guns: Fetal overnutrition and the reproduction of obesity. *Feminism & Psychology, 22*(3), 360–375.

Warin, M., Zivkovic, T., Moore, V., Ward, P. R., & Jones, M. (2015). Short horizons and obesity futures: Disjunctures between public health interventions and everyday temporalities. *Social Science & Medicine, 128*, 309–315.

Wells, J. C., Marphatia, A. A., Cole, T. J., & McCoy, D. (2012). Associations of economic and gender inequality with global obesity prevalence: Understanding the female excess. *Social Science and Medicine, 75*(3), 482–490.

World Health Organization. (2017). *Obesity*. Retrieved from http://www.who.int/topics/obesity/en/

Wright, J., & Harwood, V. (2009). *Biopolitics and the 'obesity epidemic': Governing bodies*. New York: Routledge.

Yates-Doerr, E. (2012). The opacity of reduction: Nutritional black-boxing and the meanings of nourishment. *Food, Culture and Society, 15*(2), 293–313.

Yates-Doerr, E. (2013). The mismeasure of obesity. In M. McCullough & J. Hardin (Eds.), *Reconstructing obesity: The meaning of measures and the measure of meanings* (pp. 49–70). New York: Berghahn Books.

Yates-Doerr, E. (2015). *The weight of obesity: Hunger and global health in postwar Guatemala*. Berkeley: University of California Press.

Zivkovic, T., Warin, M., Davies, M., & Moore, M. (2010). In the name of the child: The gendered politics of childhood obesity. *Journal of Sociology, 46*, 375–392.

Zivkovic, T., Warin, M., Moore, V., Ward, P., & Jones, M. (2015). The sweetness of care: Biographies, bodies and place. In E. Abbotts, A. Lavis, & L. Attala (Eds.), *Careful eating: Bodies, food and care* (pp. 109–112). Farnham: Ashgate.

CHAPTER 3

How to Taste a Trifle

We are in a food bank and Christmas is approaching. Christmas in Australia arrives in the full glare of the summer heat and, despite the weather, many families like to cook a traditional British Christmas lunch of roast meat (ham, turkey, chicken) and vegetables, followed by warm Christmas pudding and custard. The food bank workers know that Christmas can be a financial struggle for local families, and they provide a Christmas hamper for $100, which can be prepaid for in installments to ease the financial burden of the festive season. The hamper is generous and includes everything you might need for a family feast, including mince pies, biscuits, Christmas pudding, long-life custard, a whole chicken (to roast), gravy mix, bacon, mince and sausages, fresh and tinned vegetables, mixed sweets, white sugar, and long-life milk.

Christmas is thus a busy time for the food banks and local workers, making up hampers and running special cooking classes. The regular cooking class, Kids in the Kitchen, was given a festive flavor by the Obesity Prevention and Lifestyle (OPAL) workers. Designed to teach children and their parents how to cook and prepare nutritious food, the Christmas class session presented an opportunity to modify the classic dessert recipe for trifle to fit the program's health imperatives. Sugar-laden jelly crystals and sweet custard were replaced with sugar-free or low-sugar versions, banana bread substituted for sponge cake, and thick whipped cream renounced in favor of yogurt. While local staff who ran the food bank on

M. Warin, T. Zivkovic, *Fatness, Obesity, and Disadvantage in the Australian Suburbs*,
https://doi.org/10.1007/978-3-030-01009-6_3

a limited budget were disgruntled by the increased cost of these "healthy" ingredients—which they perceived as unnecessary—the icing on the cake, so to speak, was the inclusion of a range of expensive, fresh summer fruits: raspberries, blueberries, strawberries, and plums. In the words of a long-term staff member and local resident,

> I don't know why they're doing this trifle. They do not need to have so many different berries in there. It is really expensive because there's the strawberries, the blueberries, the raspberries and plums. Then there is jelly and cake. There's also custard, which is the low-fat kind, so that is expensive too. I am paying $4 just for that when you can buy the standard one here for $2.75.

"You couldn't do it for less than $20!" the worker said, aghast. Perplexed by the logic of the OPAL program and its insistence on nutritional over financial value, she tells us: "There are other things they could have done. I don't know why they aren't making gingerbread men with the kids. That is cheap and it would be a lot more fun. They could also make shortbread … it makes more sense than the trifle." Others questioned why the OPAL cooking classes did not use "home brand" (cheaper generic products) "because that's what [local customers] have to buy."

Local sensibilities of procuring food on a budget led food bank staff to purchase the raspberries a week ahead of the cooking class because they were on special (reduced price) for $8 rather than $9 a punnet. Attempts to reduce the cost of the berries failed, however, when an OPAL staff member announced that the raspberries could not be frozen. Relaying the conversation to us the food bank worker reiterated her surprise: "They need to be fresh! Really? They need to be fresh? They cost so much money!" Stuck with the costly punnets, she asked Amelia, the OPAL worker, what she should now do with all those raspberries and was baffled by her response. "She said I should sell them in the shop to the customers! But who here can afford fresh raspberries, or blueberries for that matter? Not the people who shop here." Local food bank workers and families agreed that the trifle recipe was "not very sensible." They wanted to adapt the recipe to suit local situations and finances. In the context of the food bank, the emphasis on expensive fresh raspberries was, to play on the double meaning of the term, indeed trifling.

The word trifle comes from an old French word *trufle*, and literally means something whimsical, of little consequence, or light and fluffy. Food writers trace the early origins of the dessert to the Tudor period of

Elizabethan England during which Thomas Dawson (1597) published a simple recipe made with thickened, sweetened, fragrant cream in his cookery book for the rising middle classes, *The Good Huswifes Jewell* (1597/1977). Later, embellished and widely popularized by the English cookery writer Hannah Glasse (1747/1995), the trifle took on its familiar colorful appearance with layers of cake and jelly and the inclusion of fruit, sweetmeats, and alcohol. In *The English Kitchen* series, Saberi and Davidson's (2009) book, simply entitled *Trifle*, begins by demonstrating the classed variations of the "plebeian yet aristocratic" dessert and then provides recipes adapted to suit the disparities of "cottage and castle alike" (2009, p. 11). In the course of British colonization, the trifle was improvised and transformed to suit local tastes and environments. In the USA the "Tipsy Parson" cake in the American South was made from biscuits, alcohol, and custard (and so-called for its generous quantities of sherry and popularity at church socials) while a sweet milky Indian trifle combined rice flour, cardamom, and pistachios in mid-nineteenth-century British India.

The iconic British dessert was popularized in Australia too. In recipes contributed by the local community of English and German settlers of the Barossa Valley (internationally known for its fine wine and food), which lies 40 km from our field site, *The Barossa Cookery Book* (1932) captured the versatility of the trifle in the economically depressed period of the 1930s. The Pineapple Trifle, Jelly Sponge Trifle, Cherry Trifle, Banana Trifle, and Tango Trifle, with their inclusion of canned tropical fruit and packaged custard, revealed what Santich (2012) called the Australianization of the dessert and its adaption in a "creative process not bound by prescriptive recipes" (Heuzenroeder 2006, pp. 46–49).

Indeed, these recipes are reminiscent of the trifle of our childhoods. Tanya, who grew up in public housing estates in the northern suburbs of Adelaide, recalls the trifle as the centerpiece of her grandparents' dining table on special occasions: canned (never fresh) fruit, ready-made custard, Swiss sponge cake with jam, red jelly, and cream, all colorfully assembled in a glass bowl as a dessert to enjoy after the traditional Sunday roast lunch. Like many of our fieldwork participants, Tanya's grandparents were attracted to the northern suburbs of Adelaide with their affordable housing and employment opportunities in local factories, including a thriving automotive industry. Named for Queen Elizabeth II, the satellite town was marketed as the "City for Tomorrow" and as "a place to grow," with the South Australian Government encouraging migration, particularly of

British families. Heeding the call, Tanya's grandparents, Barbara and James, arrived in 1963 with two small children on assisted passage from the UK. James quickly found work at James Hardie & Co Pty Ltd., manufacturing fibrous cement sheeting (asbestos) in their Elizabeth factory. Asbestos is the cheap, versatile (and deadly) material that enabled the rapid expansion of "fibro" homes—inexpensive dwellings that were constructed to accommodate the state's growing population of working-class UK migrant families.

We start this chapter with the British trifle as a rhetorical device, to highlight the competing ideas about food and eating, to show that even small "trifles" are indeed politically charged. In her book *Eating Culture*, Crowther (2013) similarly uses the trifle as a theoretical tool to locate the many different analyses that anthropologists might bring, and we paraphrase her at length. She asks the reader to imagine a scene in which anthropologists gather around a trifle (some, like Franz Boas who is long gone, arriving in ghostly form), each with a spoon in hand and ready to contribute their particular theoretical perspective. Boas, she says, would "approach the trifle as a particular artifact, created by historical circumstances and worthy of recording in every detail, including its recipe, manner of construction, mythological connotations, and linguistic affiliations, to preserve a record in case the trifle was lost through assimilation [or transformed through migration]" (2013, p. xvi).

As the classic ethnographer, Malinowski would be interested in the social life surrounding the trifle, calling attention to the details of the trifle's appearance, interested in "observing the scene, noting who else is appraising the trifle, and then asking participants what they understood of the trifle" (ibid., p. xxvi). Levi-Strauss would look to the trifle to "reveal deeper structures of human thought" (ibid., p. xxvii), and Mary Douglas would want to know how the trifle was positioned in the larger eating event of a meal. Hortense Powdermaker would muse on the value of trifle as a food that might be highly valued due to its capacity to enhance women's plumpness in certain historical times and cultures, and its avoidance in others due to a gendered emphasis on thinness and social status. Marshall Sahlins would assert that, due to its British origins, a cultural logic "would assign value and meaning to the trifle based on its function as a celebratory dessert with class associations" (ibid., p. xxvii). Clifford Geertz, of course, would suggest that the trifle is deeply layered with thick [custard] meaning. Arjun Appadurai would think about the trifle in terms of gastro-politics, and the trifle as a product of modernity. Sidney Mintz would focus on the sugar content and point to the ways in which the rich sweetness of the dish is imbued with colonial relations and commodity production. With a mouthful of trifle, Pierre Bourdieu would claim that preparing and eating trifle is a function of displaying taste, cultural capital, and social distinction. Carole Counihan would place gender under the spotlight and ask who made the trifle, who served it, and how its production reproduces gender relations. Johan Pottier would remind everyone that not everyone is lucky enough to eat trifle, and that issues of food security, hunger, and poverty are important backdrops (ibid., p. xxix). David Sutton would speak to the "sensual pleasures" of experiencing, in succession, "the light frothy cream, the smooth, velvety custard, the tangy fruit mingling with the bouquet of wine (or sherry or liqueur), and perhaps a touch of almondy crunchiness from ratafias or macaroons, and lastly, the sweet, soft but crumbly texture of the sponge or sponge fingers" (Saberi and Davidson 2009). And Warin (certainly not in the ilk of these esteemed anthropologists), standing back from the table with Mary Douglas, would note that there would be those who refuse to eat trifle, as people with disordered eating might consider trifle to be polluting and dirty, as too loaded with "seeping fats and flying calories" (Warin 2010).

There are indeed many ways to anthropologically "taste" a trifle. For us, there are two important aspects to highlight from this example. The first is the attention to class and taste, for the delicious layering of the sponge and custard and the cost of sweet summer berries symbolizes an indulgence laced with cultural capital and one that is not within the reach of all. Served in a glass bowl so you can see the architecture of layers, trifles are a culinary statement of taste. In his classic text *Distinction: A Social Critique of the Judgement of Taste*, Bourdieu (and other historians of food) demonstrates how taste is a marker of class, gender, and identity (Bourdieu 1984, p. 190). One's taste for certain foods, different brands of alcohol, and even the exercise one might engage in, are underpinned by *habitus*—the internalized class condition that informs our tastes and sensibilities and mediates our behaviors. Acquired over time through social conditioning and exposure to different social stimuli, *habitus* frames our personal preferences, abilities, and inclinations.

Bourdieu suggests that the concept of taste (and what constitutes "good taste" or "poor taste") is typically bourgeois (1984, p. 177). In previous work we have argued that public health interventions around food, eating, and bodies are symbolic of an idealized middle-class healthy lifestyle pattern, embodying knowledge and bodily regulation to routinely structure daily life (Warin et al. 2008, 2017).

A constant performance of taste in our fieldwork focused around the pleasures of salt, sugar, and fat. Responding to the OPAL breakfast initiative, many community members enacted local resistance to the cost, unfamiliarity, bland tastes, and implicit "goodness" of OPAL breakfast products (Warin et al. 2017). When an OPAL staff member arrived at a breakfast-themed tasting, the food bank workers suggested the vegetable frittatas needed some salt. The OPAL worker revealed how her taste preferences articulated in tune with her embodied exposures and experiences: "I just don't see the need to add salt. In my house, when I grew up, salt was never added to the food my parents cooked, so I just don't have the taste for it. I like the vegetable frittatas just the way they are." The OPAL worker understood how her own tastes have shaped her *habitus* but failed to see there could be a parallel for others. Equally, community members would not make or eat polenta for a public OPAL event, as this was considered an unfamiliar, high-brow food and not part of their everyday *habitus.*

In his discussion of taste, Bourdieu makes a distinction between tastes of luxury (freedom) and tastes of necessity. Those with an outlook of tastes of luxury are distanced from necessity in their everyday lives, forgetting the conditions that make people reach for the most filling and most economical foods (Bourdieu 1984, pp. 177–178). Taste, he says "is *amor fati*, the choice of destiny, but a forced choice, produced by condition[s] of existence which rule out all alternatives as mere daydreams and leave no choice but the taste for the necessary" (Bourdieu 1984, p. 178). Embedded in the nuances of culture, these enactments of taste permeated every interaction between OPAL staff and participants.

The trifle is useful for thinking about the place of culturally acquired taste (in Bourdieu's terms), but we do not present taste or bodies in this book as layers placed on top of each other. This is the second important point to highlight—there are hundreds of different trifle recipes. This means there are hundreds of versions, and each is prepared and eaten in different circumstances and times. For Tanya they were treats (canned and prepackaged) to end a family Sunday lunch; for others they are special desserts made "by hand and from scratch" at Christmas time. For the OPAL team they were still treats at Christmas, but healthy treats. Different versions appear in different situations.

Conceiving of trifles as versions (rather than layers) is how we approach bodies, as they "emerge and come about in different settings, practices and situations" (Mol 2012). Bodies are not like the layers of a trifle; they do not begin with a layer of the physical body that then has social layers assembled on top. Mol argues that "rather than studying piled-up *layers*" in which specialist disciplines concentrate on one layer each (starting with the biological), we may also concentrate on contrasting *versions* of the body (Mol 2012, p. 2, [her emphasis]). Versions of bodies, she argues, do not occupy a layer in a spatial pile but are events in time that emerge in different situations. Bodies are not one thing, and it is possible to differentiate between versions of the body.

We have spent some time describing how to taste a trifle, as it introduces the reader to differing conceptualizations of the body (as singular and multiple), opening a space to explore the tensions and frictions that emerged between all the different actors. Turning to the scene of the field site, the actors, and the ethnographic research process, we trace the global and local connections of the obesity program and provide a background to the history and politics of the field site location, including its position as Australia's "most adventurous postwar town planning project" (Peel 1994a, p. 36). Elizabeth was a model town designed by urban planners and settled mainly by British migrants in the 1950s.[1] We track the hopes that this area was built upon, the devastating effects of economic decline in the 1970s, and the resilience of a community that has a strong sense of, as one participant said, "being all in this together." This history is important, as the "deep and persistent disadvantage" experienced by many residents in Elizabeth led to the choosing of this site as the location for one of Australia's most ambitious obesity interventions.

Very early on in the project we remember the excitement of the OPAL staff in Adelaide as they flew to France to meet staff from the parent program called Ensemble Prévenons l'Obésité des Enfants (EPODE). The fact that a community intervention already had an international focus in Paris and across Western Europe gave a sense of importance and global momentum to the whole initiative. And being set in France, a country stereotypically known for its particular attention to cuisine and gastronomic meals (Parkhurst-Ferguson 2004, 2014), added another unspoken layer of kudos. South Australia's participation with EPODE was the first in the southern hemisphere, and everyone involved was understandably excited to be a part of this world-first program.

In the Field: Bull Ants and Heat

After not having seen him since the OPAL Festival event at Fremont Park in November, I reintroduce myself to Graham, one of the SIMPLA [Stop Income Management in Playford] organizers. "Wanna can of Coke®?" he asks. I tell him "No thanks" but he replies "C'mon, you sure?" and passes me one. I accept and feel refreshed by it in the heat, although guilty in the knowledge of its cost and my financial privilege relative to the others gathered there today. Graham lives in a suburb by the sea but spends a lot of time in Elizabeth distributing leaflets about Compulsory Income Management and SIMPLA. After I tell him that I live not far from him, he tells me "I like it out there where we are but there is something that I really like about being out here too. I might move here. I love all the open space, the trees." I agree with Graham. There are things I really like about being in Elizabeth too. The reduced council maintenance (compared to other suburbs) means that soursob flowers pop up between pavers and on council strips (and heavily adorn the front gardens of Trust housing) prettying whole streets in little yellow flowers; the rolling hills in the distance are a blanket of purple Salvation Jane [an introduced weed] and wild grasses grow tall, turning yellow and woody in summer. When it rains the smell of eucalypts bursts into the air and lingers over reddened clay terrain, settling the big bull ants who otherwise roam frenetically over the dry cracked earth. Things are less groomed, a bit more wild.

These descriptions from Tanya's field notes reveal the intimacy that being immersed in a field site can bring about. Traveling around on trains, on buses, and on foot, she noticed the cement footpaths, navigated parts of roads that were being repaired, and heard the sound of cars revving their engines as they passed. As an outer suburb of metropolitan Adelaide, Playford has an openness to spaces; things don't seem as cluttered as they do in the city and most houses don't have front fences (but a few have very high, security-laden fences with surveillance cameras). Houses built in the 1950s and 1960s are generally single-storied, with a front garden area and a garage down the side.

Approaching the main shopping centers, there are large tracts of land that are filled with native eucalypts and shrubs crisscrossed with dirt paths that wind through the scrub and lead to the shops. The houses are almost hidden behind this buffer of space. It is dry and dusty in summer, and in winter puddles of rain pool near unsheltered bus stops, and turn red. There is always someone at a bus stop, usually a mother with a few kids, one in a pram, and some grocery shopping by her side. Many of the main streets are wide and have more recently been landscaped with Australian native trees and bushes, and so the road corridors now look greener and more manicured. There aren't many traffic lights, and a main highway cuts through the city and past the ubiquitous fast food chains, providing a race track for young men in hotted-up Holden cars, flooring their accelerators as their car engines let loose a deep, guttural roar.

As you press into the different suburbs, it is easy to get lost if you are unfamiliar with landmarks. Streets wind around as boulevards, and older suburbs are focused around a small central group of shops, usually consisting of a small supermarket (a place to buy bread and milk), a post office, a video rental store, and a charity shop. Unlike the large and shiny shopping centers in the center of the town, these shops have security mesh over their windows, and roller shutters to pull down at the end of the day. In his history of the area, Peel notes how the suburbs were designed with traditional gender roles in mind—the men were the wage earners and would take the car to work in local industries, and the women (as wives and mothers) could walk to the nearby shops and have an occasional bus trip into the city center (Peel 1994b, pp. 21–22). These shops now looked tired, in need of a paint and sporting signage from years gone by. During our fieldwork they were in the process of changing, earmarked for upgrades and renovation. Renewal is very much part of local government strategy, with new housing, road upgrades, new shopping centers, and community facilities generating more local employment and pride.

People's bodies were part of this renewal agenda, not only through OPAL, but through a healthy communities' initiative from the local council. *Reshaping Playford* encouraged sustained participation of community members in healthy lifestyle programs, such as cooking classes, walking, and positive thinking. As a complementary program, OPAL was folded into and became part of the broader desire to "reshape" the residents *and* City of Playford.

A "City for Tomorrow"

The City of Playford is built on an area of Adelaide known as the Adelaide Plains. Prior to European settlement in 1836, the Kaurna Indigenous people lived on and across these lands, using traditional burning techniques to attract kangaroos and emus with the fresh growth of new grasses each season. Colonization had (and still has) devastating consequences for

Indigenous peoples across Australia; when settlers took ownership of land for farming purposes, it meant that traditional owners could no longer inhabit or move across farm lands. The Kaurna people were displaced and exposed to devastating diseases and were eventually moved into institutions and fringe-dweller camps.

Despite the thousands of years of Indigenous occupation, it is the colonist history of this area that has been extensively documented. The City of Playford has one of Australia's most interesting histories in terms of urban planning. Under the premiership of the Conservative Sir Thomas Playford (Australia's longest-serving premier, who led the state from 1938 to 1965), the South Australian State Government decided to build a British-style town north of Adelaide, based on the British "new town" concept of comprehensively planned neighborhoods (Forster and McCaskill 2007, pp. 86–87). Playford directed the South Australian Housing Trust (SAHT) (Australia's first public housing authority) to buy farmland in 1949 for the new satellite town of Elizabeth.[2]

> Elizabeth was meant to be the jewel in Liberal Premier Playford's strategy of using public planning and state subsidy to turn a state, dependent on the vicissitudes of the agricultural economy, into an industrial powerhouse. The Playford Plan was an attempt by the state to woo multinational capital from Melbourne and Sydney to Adelaide with tax breaks, cheap labour and other incentives. (Shannon 1995)

As a planned and self-contained city that was designed to be affordable, houses were inexpensive to rent, and the living costs and wages for residents were lower in Adelaide than in Sydney or Melbourne (Llewellyn-Smith 2012, p. 73).

Elizabeth was marketed as a picture-postcard place with aspirations for upward social mobility and material security. Images of white picket fences, front gardens full of roses, and men driving to work every day in shiny new cars created optimism and visions of an idealized suburban life. Brand-new affordable housing, wide suburban spaces, and secure employment through the local General Motors Holden (GMH) car industry attracted many UK working-class migrants. This new life offered people money and opportunities to secure their futures and "breathing room to keep their children in school or get them into good trades, even to take an occasional holiday" (Peel 1995a, p. 119). In the 1960s and 1970s more and more working-class UK migrant families would enact the hope that first brought them to places like Elizabeth.

British migrants contributed to a much higher percentage of Adelaide's growth than any of the other capital cities between 1947 and 1966 (Burnley 1974, cited in Marsden). The population distribution of South Australian Housing Trust tenants and house purchasers in Elizabeth was more heavily skewed to UK-born persons than Adelaide as a whole.[3] As Peel observed, British Elizabeth constituted 60 to 70 per cent of the (Elizabeth) population. In 1966, Elizabeth—not Richmond or Carlton (in Melbourne) or Leichhardt (in Sydney)—was the single most concentrated immigrant settlement in Australia (Peel 1994b, p. 20; 1995a, p. 114) (Fig. 3.1).

Not surprisingly, people who moved to Elizabeth created their own meaningful spaces in the SAHT's imagined city. There was a middle-class Elizabeth of mortgages and home owners opposed to renting tenants; "a workers' Elizabeth of worksites and an employers' Elizabeth of sites and

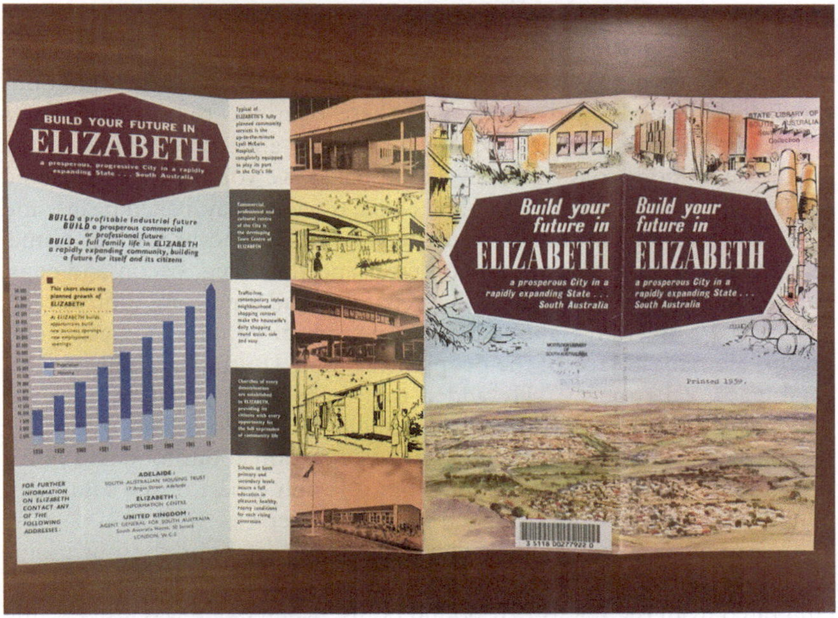

Fig. 3.1 "Build your future in Elizabeth: a prosperous city in a rapidly expanding state … South Australia." (Dates/Publication details: Adelaide: South Australian Housing Trust, 1959)

profit; a man's Elizabeth of cars, pubs, and factories and a woman's Elizabeth of streets, informal neighborhoods, and intermittent work. The model landscape splintered according to conflicting conceptions of who, and what, the town was for" (Peel 1995a, p. 56). Clearly, there were social distinctions manufactured by the SAHT planners, with a budding hierarchy of housing types and locations. Long-term residents of Playford speak about these obvious divisions, described by Peel as "boundaries based on class, with carefully delineated divisions between types of housing and the types of residents expected to inhabit them" (Peel 1995a, p. 51). The flat "pancake" plains were designated for rental housing and the low-slung hills behind were the "high country" or "middle-class hill slopes" intended to "provide a better class residential area as the town developed" (Peel 1995a, p. 48). Often, it was high-ranking employees of the nearby Royal Australian Air Force base who were given superior accommodation (ibid.). These divisions are still apparent, with our participants describing some parts of Elizabeth as "flashy," whereas other areas were described as "no go zones" or "Crazy Town."

During the 1950s and 1960s, the foods that were enjoyed by Playford residents (and white Australians more widely) were based on the traditions the British brought with them, and these continue to have resonance today (despite the greater diversity of cultures and cuisines now in the area). Many foods sold in the two food banks we volunteered in catered for this palate, selling frozen fish and chips, tuna mornay, baked beans, and Shepherd's Pie. When asked what they like to eat and prepare at home, many people said they liked to eat "meat and three veg, bacon and eggs, bangers and mash." One day while preparing salad for a community event, Colin talked to Tanya about his experiences of running a local men's group. He said: "Many of the people who come [to the men's group] eat total crap, real rubbish." He added that many of the men "don't even know what the names of different vegetables are let alone how to prepare them." Based on this he thinks that basic education about food and nutrition is important in the community, but it is only a part of the solution if communities are to be encouraged to be healthier.

Colin says that his family did not think much about the nutritional value of food when he was growing up. His parents are Scots and they all emigrated from the UK as "10-pound poms" when Colin was just a young boy. "We used to eat fatty meat, really unhealthy, and we'd eat a lot of it. It was always meat and veg but then when I was around 13 I got my first girlfriend and she was Maltese. I'd never had any exposure at all to other cultures and so when I went around to her house and there was all of this fantastic food to eat I couldn't believe it: I was in heaven!" Colin tells Tanya though that this is not always the experience for people who come to Australia as 10-pound poms: "I've met men here who have never tried rice, or never eaten pasta and when you ask why they haven't tried pasta they'll say, 'That's wog[4] food—I'm not eating wog food'." Colin feels that the strong concentration of English migrants in the Playford area has contributed to a conservative food culture where "meat and three veg" is often seen as the standard diet.

The food banks, however, did reflect a gradual shift in food cultures. They stocked chow mein, fried rice, chicken stir-fry, and spaghetti bolognaise meal packs alongside more typically English fare, and at the time of our fieldwork staff were beginning to receive (and wondering how to respond to) questions about halal foods from newly arrived East African families.

In their analysis of the changing eating and food habits of Australians across three generations, Banwell et al. (2012) note that "in economically restricted times [families were] brought up to view food pragmatically, focusing on its cost and its ability to keep the family from feeling hungry" (2012, p. 24). This practical attitude is also influenced by the dominant sociocultural perspective on food, reflecting Australia's history as an English colony (Symons 2007; Walker and Roberts 1988). This was especially the case in Elizabeth, where residents were reliant on a manufacturing economy that has been subject to market deregulation (and subsequent decline in employment) over the last 40 years.

Rising rates of obesity in Australia from the early 2000s turned the attention of dieticians to lower socioeconomic locales, noting the higher incidence of overweight and obesity in areas of disadvantage, and the perceived lack of knowledge of nutrition and healthy eating. This set the scene for well-intentioned public health interventions to operate in the community, and the next section focuses on how a 'City for Tomorrow' became the "territory of the battler" (Peel 1995b, p. 131), and identification as a key location for OPAL.

Pockets of "Deep and Persistent Disadvantage"

Mark Peel describes Elizabeth as "a place made poor" (1994a). He remembers Elizabeth as once a "decent place to live, a place for projects and aspirations, where successes outweighed failures" (1994a, p. 37). He makes a strong case in arguing that it was not the assumed high concentration of working-class families that created a "social problem," but the state's economic crisis which stripped the area of its jobs and resources and led to a shrinking public sector. During the 1970s the car industry began to fail and retrenchments took place at GMH and also at the factories that supplied them with automotive parts. Once employing 7000 workers (men and women and half of them local residents), the industry cut thousands of jobs. The effects of unemployment and cutbacks were seen in new buildings (a new courthouse and a new police station), and also in "crumbling schools and declining services" (Peel 1994a, p. 36).

The role of the SAHT also dramatically changed during this time. Conservative Australian politics led to severe funding cuts, and "slashing for slashing's sake became the dominant policy option in welfare and housing" (Peel 1995a, p. 185). The Trust became known not as an organization providing low-cost housing for working families, but as a welfare agency that provided welfare housing:

> Elizabeth's compact rental estates filled with the unemployed victims of recession and with new groups of stigmatized welfare beneficiaries like single mothers. Within public housing estates, divisions emerged between older long-term tenants, often retired or widowed, and the groups making up the so-called new poor. (Peel 1995a, pp. 188–189)

Elizabeth was not alone in its decline during the 1970s recession. Estates in Britain also witnessed a savage polarization between "those who are given, and take, the opportunity to adjust to a lifetime of insecure, shifting or intensified employment, and those who do not even get that chance" (Peel 1995a, p. 195). Steel working cities, like Fontana in California and Wollongong in Australia, suffered similar fates. Following the downturn, all of these cities faced an "uncertain future" (Peel 1995a, p. 156).

Despite the significant recent investment in urban regeneration projects and new housing developments in Elizabeth and surrounding suburbs, what was heralded as the City for Tomorrow in government brochures of the 1960s today remains a place that has pockets of *Deep and Persistent Disadvantage* (McLachlan et al. 2013)[5] and at the time of our fieldwork had the nation's second-highest youth unemployment rate of 41%. Households are characterized by low incomes, and a disproportionate number of people have poor health and/or a disability, requiring assistance with core activities of daily living. Almost 40% of children under the age of 16 live in low-income, welfare-dependent households (Hordacre et al. 2013). Three percent of people identify as Indigenous (greater than the state as a whole at 1.9%) and 27% were born outside Australia (mostly in England or Scotland). In recent years the area has welcomed more than 2000 migrants—half from the humanitarian stream, the most disadvantaged of migrants, many of whom came from southern and eastern Africa (Hordacre et al. 2013, p. v).

It was often stressed by council staff and some participants that this adversity generated a strong sense of pride and a strong sense of community. This pride had a temporal dimension and was leveraged to bolster people's hope. We found, however, that horizons were short and many participants had difficulty imagining their futures. Temporality was experienced through "the here and now," "one day at a time," or "today and tomorrow and next week." Angela, a volunteer in the food bank, said: "People come in here just thinking of now, the moment, the next meal, maybe even the next couple of days but not beyond that."

This future discounting impacted people's drive to change present behaviors to mitigate future health risks (Warin et al. 2015). Ellie, a socially isolated, unemployed 63-year-old woman, captured how decisions were made according to either future health or immediate pleasures:

> "Life's tough. A couple of months ago my doctor diagnosed me with chronic obstructive pulmonary disease. I lose my breath if I do anything quickly. It's the cigarettes. My doctor says I'd live another 5 years if I gave up smoking," Ellie says, shrugging her shoulders and huffing "Pah! Another five years! I don't really know if I'd want that. Another five years. Of this?" A weary expression creeps across her face. "But you know I could do with a bit more money, so I've cut down. I worked it out. You see I buy packets of 40 and each cigarette is a little more than 50 cents so by smoking eight cigarettes less a day I'm saving $4. It all adds up. But why would I stop? Really, what do I have in my life? Nothing. This is my only pleasure in life."

The health of the people in this community is directly linked to successive decades of economic decline and social disadvantage. As we detailed in Chap. 1, obesity is more prevalent among families living in this community than in the general population, but this did not necessarily mean that it was a particular concern or focus for families. More important was the capacity to financially support oneself and one's family, fill stomachs with food (what Mol refers to as "the belly feeling" (2012, p. 9)) and pay the bills.

Most participants involved in our project lived in difficult circumstances. Many had chronic health conditions (depression, diabetes, chronic pain) and would be deemed to be overweight or obese according to body mass index (BMI) measures. Of the community members we interviewed only two were employed in full-time work, and seven had part-time work (some ongoing but most short term). The majority (80%) were on welfare payments (Austudy, Carer Allowance, Newstart, Parenting Payment), including disability pensions and the aged pension. Welfare payments varied according to family circumstances (if you lived alone or had children), but on average, a weekly welfare payment for a sole parent with dependent children was about A$ 295. This is about A$ 40 a day.

During our fieldwork (in July 2012) Place-Based Income Management began in Australia, a program targeting communities that were identified as vulnerable. This involved a five-year trial to "manage" household finances in five socially disadvantaged communities across Australia, including one in South Australia (which happened to be our field site). Welfare recipients in Playford could choose to become income-managed and, in certain circumstances, compulsory income management could be enforced by the state. Compulsory income management can occur when welfare recipients are referred for Child Protection Income Management by state child protection authorities, or selected for the Vulnerable Welfare Payment after being assessed as vulnerable to financial crisis, or if they qualify for the Disengaged Youth Measure, which applies to young people between the ages of 15 and 25 who have been on government benefits for 13 weeks or longer. Income management in the new place-based policy involves the quarantining of 50–70% of government welfare benefits for direct debit of essential household expenses (rent, bills, education, medical costs). Income-managed funds could also be accessed by a Basics Card for the purchase of basic living expenses, such as food and clothing purchased from designated retailers. The Basics Card, however, was not accepted at fast food outlets, nor could it be used to purchase prohibited items, such as drugs, alcohol, cigarettes, gambling, or pornography.

In a local contribution to the state government consultation *An Affordable Place To Live*, community members in Playford described income management as having "a destructive effect on families," as it prioritized the cost of housing and children, "resulting in some parents going without meals, cutting back on the weekly shopping, or foregoing fresh fruit and vegetables" (Uniting Communities and Community Centres SA 2013). These unintended consequences of income management underscored increased financial pressure on poor families as they tried to make money and food stretch from one pay to the next.

Participants in our study described pay weeks as "on weeks" or "good weeks" that were characterized by increased food intake, contrasting with "off weeks" or "bad weeks," when food intake was constrained by limited budgets. In "bad weeks" skipping meals or going days without food formed part of a deliberate financial strategy, as in the case of 44-year-old John, who explained how living healthily was something that was very difficult to do if you were unemployed. "Food is the first thing that drops off. I mean you gotta pay your rent and your bills or you'll end up without a place to live." John lives on a limited government allowance of less than $315 a week, $200 of which he pays in rent. With rising costs of living and no proportionate increase in government benefits, John can only spend $10 a fortnight on public transport (the equivalent of two days travel), cannot run or reregister his car, and can spend no more than $50 a fortnight on food and other household items. "I enjoy my food," John says as he explains how he'd like to have a varied diet of fruit, veg, meat, and dairy, but when an unforeseen expense arises, and they often do, he'll go without meals or live for days, even weeks, on bread and butter because, he says: "If I've got no money, I gotta get by the cheapest way I can."

Local responses to income management in Playford were varied. While some people wanted to have their income managed and volunteered for it (in part for the $250 incentive to sign up to the scheme) others were opposed to the policy, claiming it to be "disempowering," "a breach of welfare rights," and "ineffective" since, as one participant said, "problems such as substance abuse run so much deeper than money." Social worker Mendes critiqued the policy for taking an individualistic interpretation of social disadvantage which, he said, "tends to assume that people are poor or unemployed [or substance dependent] because of behavioral characteristics such as incompetence, immortality or laziness" (2013, p. 495). Turning the tables on the epithet often ascribed to them in local media and in popular stereotypes of Adelaide's northern suburbs, some welfare recipients in Playford condemned compulsory income management as being a "lazy policy" because it did not address the underlying structural issues of poverty and unemployment in which their lives were embedded.

Community meetings and demonstrations organized by a resistance group to income management in Playford provided a forum for local people to protest against the welfare reform, raise concerns about the techniques of surveillance that operated to "refer" them for compulsory income management, and share their day-to-day experiences of living on benefits. Stop Income Management in Playford (SIMPLA) events were sometimes held in conjunction with the Single Parents Action Group (SPAG). Founded by local single mums, SPAG began in response to government spending cuts to single parents' income by moving them off of the single-parent benefit and onto Newstart, which forced parents to actively seek employment and engage in unpaid "mutual obligation" activities, such as voluntary work, for 15 hours a week. A common sentiment expressed in these meetings was increasing financial hardship for welfare recipients and strident resistance to being managed in such a paternalistic and punitive manner. It is in this context and into this political climate that OPAL was introduced to and operated in the community.

Introducing OPAL: A French Twist

In 2008 the Labor State Health Minister of South Australia John Hill visited France and learned about a community program tackling obesity. In the memoir of his political career, Hill highlights the importance of illness prevention, and how he became an enthusiast (2016, p. 77) for an obesity prevention program that Jean-Michel Borys had established in France. Borys was a French doctor (trained in endocrinology) who worked in the working-class town of Beauvais in the suburbs north of Paris. Hill recounts that Borys had become concerned about the incidence of heart disease among his patients and had started to have success with a "social-change-focused approach, involving children, families, schools, community and local government" (ibid.). This social change program was called EPODE.

EPODE was based on the earlier Fleurbaix-Laventie Ville Santé study, a school-based nutrition information program that began in 1992 and was based in the northern French towns of Fleurbaix and Laventie. The intervention to prevent overweight in children preceded a number of other community-based initiatives, including walk to school days, organized family activities, the building of new sporting facilities, and the employment of sports educators (Romon et al. 2009, p. 1736). It has been estimated that 80% of the towns' populations were actively involved in the community initiative (Westley 2007). A 12-year longitudinal study of the intervention determined a reversal in weight gain among the campaign target group. By 2005 the prevalence of childhood overweight had declined by 8.8% in sharp contrast to the 17.8% rise in the study's two comparison towns (Katan 2009, p. 924). The researchers concluded that over sustained periods "interventions targeting a variety of population groups can have synergistic effects on overweight prevalence" (Romon et al. 2009, p. 1735). The success of the campaign has been attributed to community commitment to the program and to its expansion beyond schools to include and engage with many stakeholders including general practitioners, pharmacists, dieticians, shopkeepers, cultural and sporting facilities, families, and town councilors (Romon et al. 2009, p. 1736).

It was on the back of the success of the Fleurbaix-Laventie Ville Santé study that Borys initiated the community-based obesity prevention campaign EPODE. EPODE began in France in January 2004 and the community-based methodology was developed by Proteines (a French advertising company) (c.f. Hartwick 2014, p. 67). Proteines produced stylish marketing around the EPODE campaign and considering the lack of success with any global obesity intervention study, there was a lot of hype around this one's potential. It was initially rolled out in ten towns, and the intervention has since spread to over 100 French communities and has generated similar programs in Europe, Central America, and Australia. Borys is now the director of the EPODE European Network (Borys et al. 2012).

In EPODE a target group of children in an age range of 5–12 years are measured and weighed annually to determine their BMI. Interviews are conducted by school doctors who provide parents with letters about the health of their children and information on nutrition and physical exercise. Children deemed to be overweight or at risk of being so are encouraged to see a doctor. Community members can design and implement their own initiatives after their submissions are approved by a central committee. Activities involved in EPODE include leaflet distribution, classroom education about vegetables, and organizing safe routes for walking to school. At the time there were no systematic or conclusive evaluations of the EPODE campaign but preliminary findings suggested a significant decrease in the prevalence of overweight and obesity between 2005 and 2007 (Westley 2007).[6]

John Hill was so impressed with EPODE that he invited Borys to Australia, with the explicit aim of introducing a similar scheme in South Australia. Bipartisanship across all levels of government and industry involvement were seen to be key to the success of the French program, and in his desire to model this success in South Australia, Hill arranged for

Borys to make a presentation in Adelaide to the South Australian parliament. Some ministers (from all sides of government) were similarly enthused; however, the push to involve industry partners as had occurred in France (such as with Nestlé) was viewed as a major conflict of interest by others. As a result, bipartisanship between Conservative and Labor factions was unsuccessful (Hill 2016, p. 76).

EPODE's involvement with certain industries continued to be a sticking point and was used by the then shadow Education Minister David Pisoni to call into question the links between a healthy eating program and the fast food industry. Pisoni claimed that the South Australian Labor Government "has been caught out by the spin doctors of the junk food industry" (2008a). Pisoni was highly suspicious because EPODE was sponsored by Nestlé®, the French sugar industry, and pharmaceutical and artificial sweetener manufacturers. Borys was also the director of the Proteines agency, which marketed EPODE—an advertising company whose clients included McDonald's®, Coca Cola®, and Ferrara® (the latter company famously known for running advertisements about the health benefits of a chocolate spread). In his own research to provide evidence of the supposed dubious links of the French program, Pisoni found that Borys had written a paper on the benefits of drinking beer, which was funded by Brewers of Europe (Benefits of Moderate Beer Consumption 2002). One of the key points from this report, Pisoni claimed, was that beer can make a positive contribution to a healthy diet as it is made from "wholesome ingredients," provides essential vitamins and minerals, and is healthy: "Beer is 93% water and is an enjoyable means of taking this essential substance. Beer is a thirst quenching long drink which is relatively low in alcohol" (Pisoni 2008a). Seeing through what he considered as the self-interest of corporate sponsorship, Pisoni sought to discredit such claims by publicly airing his opinion to the media: "What the Minister won't tell us is what credibility test he did on the doctor who claims that drinking beer is an effective way of drinking water" (Pisoni 2008b).

Criticisms of EPODE were also raised by academics.[7] Daniel, Paquet, and McDermott (2009) voiced their concerns about the evaluation of the Fleurbaix–Laventie study conducted by Romon and colleagues in 2008, a study that was said to underpin the EPODE methodology. In a letter to the editor of the journal *Public Health Nutrition* in 2009 they pointed to the poorly described evidence base of the French intervention study, highlighting significant gaps in their approach to planning, and the measurement of change, stating that "[i]n this study, the nature of the intervention components was not adequately described, nor the 'dose(s)', nor how community structures facilitated implementation, penetration, and uptake of the intervention components" (2009, p. 1306). Daniel, Paquet, and McDermott (2009) stated that the details of the study were confusing, and concluded by asking the following:

> Given the potential significance of this study as a model for multi-level solutions to obesity among youth, and potential assumptions about the causal basis of its effects, we ask the authors to respond and also to publish a more detailed description to enable a transparent assessment of the intervention, basis for inference on its results and potential generalisability elsewhere. (2009, p. 1306)

Despite the lack of bipartisan support and academic criticisms of prior program evaluation, EPODE continued to be touted as a success and was brought to South Australia. The timing was right in terms of government support for new public health projects (including the establishment of the Australian National Preventive Health Agency (ANPHA) in 2011), as it was obvious that the traditional obesity prevention programs that simply instructed people to eat less or exercise more had not resulted in an overall reduction of BMI. Academics and practitioners were arguing that obesity prevention required a multifaceted approach (Economos and Irish-Hauser 2007; Flynn et al. 2006; Peterson and Fox 2007; Summerbell et al. 2009; Swinburn and de Silva-Sanigorski 2010). Often these directives called for multi-strategy, multi-setting prevention, community-wide interventions, and capacity building, so that "long-term results may be achieved through ongoing support from society as a whole, including parents, schools, and government agencies" (Romon et al. 2009, p. 1741).

South Australia Health paid an initial license agreement fee to Proteines of \$653,070 over four years, from 2009 to 2012, to establish EPODE in South Australia (Hansard 2013). Phase 1 commenced in 2009 and included four local metropolitan council areas (City of Marion, City of Onkaparinga, City of Playford, City of Salisbury) and two regional areas (City of Mount Gambier and City of Port Augusta). According to the OPAL Guidebook (2012, p. 56), areas were selected according to these criteria:

- Population equaling somewhere around 10,000–30,000
- Low socioeconomic status—those in greatest need
- High levels of overweight and obesity

- High proportion/number of children
- Recognized communities—geographically linked
- Existing infrastructure (services, e.g. schools, childcare, food supply, staff)

The name Obesity Prevention and Lifestyle (OPAL) was chosen by Minister John Hill. He was given a short list of possible acronyms to choose from and instructed that the acronym needed to "stand alone" but also have the word obesity in it. This was a requirement by EPODE as it was seen as a political imperative to have obesity in the name (in terms of funding) but the minister also wanted a name that could be used within the community ("OPAL") without using the word obesity. When John Hill selected OPAL from the list, it was an opportunity to draw in his friend Rachael Sporn (Olympic medal winner from the Australian women's national basketball team called the Opals) who would act as a role model for the OPAL program. Rachael, who was appointed Deputy Chair of the OPAL Scientific Strategic Advisory Committee in the early days, would take her medals to some primary schools to talk with children about being active and eating well for OPAL.

The Fleurbaix-Laventie Ville Santé study and EPODE was cited in the OPAL branding as a "globally proven model" (Guidebook 2012, p. 32) and was always used to legitimate the introduction of OPAL in South Australia. It provided a backdrop that was credible, as the success of the program was always highlighted, and again, the unstated distinction of the French to be international leaders in food and eating was almost unquestionable. If anyone knew about food and eating, it was the French.

OPAL was introduced to stakeholders in South Australia by way of a familiar narrative. It began with "A Tale of Two French Towns," as the City of Playford website highlights:

> When the two French towns of Fleurbaix and Laventie showed that a whole-of-community approach could have a major impact on turning around childhood obesity, South Australia was ready to know more.
>
> The French program, called EPODE (translated as "together we can prevent childhood obesity"), found that childhood obesity in the two pilot towns did not increase, while in two comparison towns, where there was no community-wide lifestyle program, obesity levels doubled.
>
> Children in the EPODE towns also had a better knowledge of nutrition, had made major changes to their eating habits, and had increased their phys-

> ical activity. The French approach found that the key to success was involving the whole community—families, local GPs, pharmacists, shop owners, local government, sports and cultural associations, as well as schools.
>
> Now run in over 250 communities throughout Europe, the success of this community-based approach was too strong to ignore.

The effectiveness of the program was presented as persuasive and compelling. The next step in the logic was to identify a problem in South Australia:

> Amongst 4-year-olds in South Australia, nearly one in five is overweight or obese, and more than half of South Australia's adults are overweight or obese. Being overweight can affect the physical, emotional, and social well-being of children. Overweight children are very likely to become overweight adults, with a greatly increased risk of heart disease, type-2 diabetes and other chronic health problems.

This follows the pattern of discourse identified in the previous chapter: a classic Foucauldian trajectory in which a problem is identified and discursively constructed, evidence collected to support the weight of the problem (in this case through epidemiological data), the consequences of not addressing the problem (co-morbidities), the economic costs of the problem, and finally a solution to the problem—OPAL—put forward. It was intended that OPAL would build on the European success story, working with a range of communities to positively change attitudes and behaviors about healthy eating and physical activity. The table was set, and the required accoutrements (manuals, social marketing props of posters, brochures, drink bottles, and lunch box tags) identified and set in motion. It was these heterogeneous elements of people, events, and objects that were tied together into the material and conceptual order of a successful project (Latour 2000)—imagined as "the jewel in our health crown" (Playford Community Newsletter 2012).

"Reshaping" Playford

In her study of how a French model of obesity prevention was transferred to South Australia, Hartwick (2014) notes the vastly different cultural environments between France and Australia, specifically in terms of their food and lifestyle habits (2014, p. 276). There are, she suggests major differences in terms of "food models, physical activity habits, parenting methods and education strategies in community, school and family environments" (ibid.).

France is well served by a government that strives to maintain the distinctiveness of its food and production through tight policies, regulations, and laws. Food and food rituals in French culture are so highly valued that in 2010 the United Nations Educational, Scientific and Cultural Organization (UNESCO) declared that the French gastronomic meal fulfilled the conditions for being a "world intangible heritage." There are sections of the French community that are deeply resistant to globalization, including the spread of genetically modified foods (Sato 2013), and the Americanization of food, with the French Government banning the use of American condiments like ketchup in school cafeterias. Despite the high number of McDonald's® outlets in France, there have been many local sites of resistance to such Americanization of eating. Perhaps the most famous act of public resistance was performed by José Bové, a French sheep farmer and activist, who, in 1999, gained fame overnight by leading an attack on a partially constructed McDonald's in his town. The attack was motivated by a trade war with America, and the subsequent surcharge on the highly valued French cheese Roquefort (Bové and Dufour 2002). Bové was sentenced for his attack, and, in defiance (and with support from French sociologist Pierre Bourdieu), drove his tractor in a seven-hour procession from his farm near Millau in southwest France to a jail near Montpellier, 97 kms away, where he was imprisoned for three months.

The French Government plays a strong interventionist role in relation to health and nutrition. The French national nutrition and health program (Programme National Nutrition Santé [PNNS]) began in 2001 and is a long-term public health initiative that focuses on improving the nutrition and health status of the French population. This is a nationwide program that identifies education and information as a key strategy to influence food behaviors, but also understands nutrition quite broadly in terms of foods, social determinants, cultural, economic, sensorial, and cognitive aspects of food practices (Sanabria 2015, p. 5). The PNNS is designed to protect French culture:

> The national nutrition and health program (PNNS) is a public health policy led by the Ministry of Health linked with the ministries in charge of agricultural, consumption, social cohesion, national education, sports and youth, research and local government. (Bertrand 2006, cited in Hartwick 2014, p. 291)

In terms of obesity, the PNNS considers childhood obesity to be a societal issue, a public health issue, and the responsibility of the French Government to intervene (Hartwick 2014, p. 291).

Australia has a very different set of cultural mores when it comes to food consumption and national identity. There is great diversity in Australian foods, which reflects the increasing diversity of settled migrants, especially after the dismantling of the White Australia Policy in 1973. Following the postwar waves of British, Greek, and Italian migrants, Australia's culinary landscape has more recently flourished due to Asian influences from China, Vietnam, Indonesia, and Malaysia. While "fusion foods" are now familiar to some Australian palates, barbeques, steak, fish and chips, and meat pies continue to cling on as traditional favorites (Alonso and Krajsic 2016). Sadly, there has been little regard for Indigenous foods, and despite Aboriginal people living off the land for thousands of years, any respect for Indigenous land use, land care, and food provision was long ago dismissed in favor of European agricultural management (see Santich 2011).

As well as *what* we eat, Hartwick notes that *how* we eat has changed. In contrast to French norms, "Australian foodways have become characterized by a lack of structure or rules" (Hartwick 2014, p. 77). Venn et al. (2017) chart the changing eating habits of Australians across recent decades, citing "destructured dining" (or what Poulain refers to as "vagabond eating" (2002)) as one of many possible reasons for diet-related health risks such as obesity. In addition, other factors, such as greater cultural diversity, changing work patterns, and household composition, play a role in changing diets and how, where, and what people eat.

Unlike France, Australia does not have a national policy or program to address nutrition or obesity. The political climate in Australia is underpinned by a neoliberal ideology which rejects any perceived measures to model a "nanny state." In a free market economy, individuals are thus expected to take responsibility for their own health. This is best exemplified by Australian Government ministers who tell Australians that in order to "fix the obesity problem" all we need to do is "push back from the table," "cut back on the number of chocolate milk cartons we drink per day," or undergo gastric surgery.

Public health has always struggled to compete with biomedical sciences and tertiary care in Australia. Labor governments have had better success at promoting the clear economic and societal benefits of health promotion, as seen in the 1970s Whitlam era that ushered in community health centers. In 2008, under a Labor government, the National Partnership Agreement on Preventive Health (NPAPH) was announced by the Council of Australian Governments (COAG). This is around the time that John Hill was successful in bringing EPODE to Australia. The NPAPH was the largest investment ever made by an Australian Government in health prevention. In 2012 funds were allocated through the ANPHA to projects that addressed the rising prevalence of lifestyle-related chronic disease (obesity, tobacco, and alcohol) by laying the foundations for healthy behaviors in the daily lives of Australians through community settings such as childcare centers, schools, and workplaces, supported by national social marketing campaigns. In 2013, when the pendulum swung back and a coalition (Liberal–National Party) government was elected, the NPAPH and ANPHA were immediately axed in the first budget (and OPAL's funding was severely cut).

Another major contrast in French and Australian cultural practices concerns the role of schools in educating about food. In France, the national education system entirely controls what children eat during the day and plays a major role in protecting and maintaining French culture and culinary tradition (Hartwick 2014, p. 295). In school each day, French children enjoy a "nutritionally balanced sit-down meal at lunch time," and are taught about the pleasures of taste, table etiquette, and conviviality.

In Australia, primary school children have a very different experience. They are not provided with a balanced, hot sit-down meal. Instead, they take a lunch box from home (usually consisting of a sandwich, some snacks, and/or fruit) and are allocated a brief period (on average ten minutes) to sit in their classrooms and eat before going to play outside for the rest of the lunch break. Penny, a community education officer at a local primary school, summed up the routine: "In schools now, well, at our school, the kids eat inside, inside the classroom from 1 pm until 1.10." Tanya asked why they eat inside. Penny elaborated:

> I think it's because of bullying and peer pressure; it also stops kids from swapping lunches, or at least it's meant to, but you should see some of the stuff that still goes on, what some of the kids eat for lunch each day. Sometimes it breaks your heart to see what some of the kids bring to school. One kid brings in a whole packet of biscuits each day, the "shit" biscuits, those ones from Cheap as Chips—you can imagine \$1 a packet and [the parent] gives the kids the same packet every day. I mean it's difficult in that no matter how right you get the policy and how right you get the schools, like, if the policy and the schools are on board with healthy eating and the

kids are being taught about nutrition, it might not be enough. It all depends on what else is going on, like at home with the parents and what they are eating and the access to food that they have.

Most Australian primary schools have canteens, which offer a range of "healthy" and "non-healthy" options, depending on the school's policy and governance. Children are often allowed to snack during the day at school, whereas in France the morning snack was deemed unnecessary by the PNNS program and snacking between meals is actively discouraged. Here there is no specific focus on food and the sensory pleasures of eating as there is in France, and the idea of sitting down at tables with knives and forks and eating three courses—a main meal, a salad, and a piece of fruit, as French school children do—is far removed from Australian cultural practices.[8]

Interestingly (and as Hartwick also notes), French cultural food principles were not overtly included in the EPODE "methodology,"[9] which has the following four "pillars":

- A strong political will, thanks to the support of political representatives
- Coordinated organizational systems based on social marketing methods
- A multi-level, multi-stakeholder approach, involving both public and private partners
- Sound scientific basis for evaluation, and dissemination of the program

It is surprising that the cultural principles of food and eating, which were central to EPODE, were not included among these central pillars. Hartwick suggests that this was because food practices are so taken for granted and so embedded in France that they were overlooked (Hartwick 2014, p. 310). Taste, pleasure, and conviviality are so much a part of the French food culture that perhaps it was too obvious to restate.[10]

Similarly, in Australia, OPAL was not linked to any Australian food culture, and there was no emphasis on taste or food appreciation. In fact, Australia "deliberately discarded the food principles at the foundation of EPODE" (Hartwick 2014, p. 305). Rather, the emphasis was on a science-based approach to health, nutrition (ibid., p. 305), and physical activity in which food was characterized as either "good" or "bad." The social importance of food was rarely mentioned when OPAL was promoted in Playford.

In summing up the differences in the transposing of EPODE to OPAL, Hartwick characterizes the French program as reinforcing cultural values, and the Australian program as introducing new ideas. So in France, the EPODE program *reinforced* existing supports and was intimately linked with the French food culture. In Australia, the OPAL program played a role of change agent, aiming to *introduce new attitudes* and to increase community knowledge around healthy foods and healthy lifestyles (Hartwick 2014, p. 287).

* * *

In this chapter we have examined the entanglements of place and taste that came to bear on the OPAL program. Like the layers of a trifle, we have assembled the history of Elizabeth and traced its optimistic beginnings and its struggles since the 1970s. In order to grasp the politics at play, it is important to know this history, as it is key to understanding the struggles and pride that constitute daily lives. This hardship was important to constructions of personhood (being "from the northern suburbs") but was also actively downplayed in the OPAL program. Downplaying local experiences of hardship meant that tensions began to arise behind the scenes. People questioned the costs of all the OPAL social marketing posters and brochures. Renata, a food bank volunteer, pointed to the OPAL posters and pamphlets that lined the walls of the food bank and asked: "Does all that government funding actually end up feeding kids or does it go on this marketing and these posters?" Others questioned the supposed ease of changing eating habits. When local people complained that buying fresh fruit and vegetables was too expensive, OPAL staff worked hard to challenge this "myth," saying "[f]ruit and veg is really not that expensive when you compare it to processed foods." A young mother of two disagreed. "Last week the apples were, like, $4 a kilo. That is pretty expensive if you ask me." A different community member in the group said: "It all depends on where you buy them from."

Like the trifle that we started this chapter with, there were many versions of health, eating, and bodies at play in our fieldwork. And each version had a different register of value (Heuts and Mol 2013). Some registers were about affordability, others about tastes and pleasures, the capacity to plan ahead, practices of care, and what constitutes "good health." There were tensions between and within these registers that led to clashes and compromises. Often these registers shifted from one situation to another and according to the social relationships and places in which they emerged. The questions we turn to in the next chapter are how OPAL accounted for these differing registers, and which version of health this program ultimately embraced.

Notes

1. South Australia does differ significantly in history from the other Australian states as it was not settled by English convicts or with convict labor. In 1834 the South Australia Colonization Act was passed in Britain to establish a free-settler colony, granting a huge swathe of land to new settlers who came with the desire to establish a democratic, British model of society.
2. The City of Playford was established in 1997, an amalgamation of the cities of Elizabeth and Munno Para.
3. Susan Marsden notes that British migrants expected to have rights to public housing "compared to the attitudes of Greek and Italian settlers, who had a higher propensity to purchase houses" (www.sahistorians.org.au/175/bm.doc/playfords-metroplis-2.doc)
4. "Wog" is Australian slang for Mediterranean migrants, predominantly Italians who came to Australia in the 1950s. It has more recently been taken up by Greek and Italian Australians as a self-identifying term, resulting in disempowerment of the racist overtones it once held.
5. Although individual postcodes were not identified in the written report, the outer northern suburb of Elizabeth in the City of Playford was clearly identified in national media releases by the authors.
6. A study examining five different communities that implemented EPODE found that "although the implementation of the initial EPODE program led to promising results, similar Intersectoral community Approach towards Childhood Obesity (IACO)s have shown significantly less impact on health-related outcomes" (van der Kleij et al. 2016, p. 99).
7. From interviews with members of OPAL's Scientific Advisory Committee and the Strategic Advisory Committee, Louise Townend similarly highlights reservations that were held about EPODE's evaluation and success: "They actually didn't have much in—virtually no evaluation (Rose)." "I felt that … EPODE was perhaps suggesting a strategy that had not been evaluated as effective" (Ben) (2015, p. 170).
8. The Australian Stephanie Alexander Kitchen Garden program, which promotes the pleasures of food in education, is an exception to this (https://www.kitchengardenfoundation.org.au/).

9. It is unusual that these pillars are described as "methodologies." In research a methodology is the particular research design that guides the researcher in choosing methods, for example experimental research, action research, or ethnography (Crotty 1998, pp. 1–5). The pillars described by EPODE and OPAL are a mixture of different approaches, not methodologies.
10. In her ethnographic work on obesity in France, Emilia Sanabria explores the Research Group on Overweight and Obesity (GROS—literally fat/big) who engage in "therapeutic education that is centred on the eater's bodily sensations" (Sanabria 2015, p. 126). In this program, "pleasure is a leitmotif" (ibid.).

References

Alonso, A., & Krajsic, V. (2016). Perceptions and images of 'typical Australian dishes': An exploratory study. *Journal of Foodservice Business Research, 19*(2), 147–163.

Banwell, C., Broom, D., Davies, A., & Dixon, J. (2012). From habit to choice: Transformations in family dining over three generations. In *Weight of modernity: An intergenerational study of the rise of obesity* (pp. 23–39). Dordrecht: Springer.

Bertrand, X. (2006). *Deuxième Programme national nutrition santé (PNNS)*. Paris: Ministère de la Santé et des Solidarités.

Borys, J. M., Le Bodo, Y., Jebb, S. A., et al. (2012). EPODE approach for childhood obesity prevention: Methods, progress and international development. *Obesity Reviews, 13*(4), 299–315.

Bourdieu, P. (1984). *Distinction: A social critique of the judgment of taste* (trans: Nice, R.). Cambridge: Harvard University Press.

Bové, J., & Dufour, F. (2002). *The world is not for sale: Farmers against junk food*. London: Verso.

Brewers of Europe. (2002). *Benefits of moderate beer consumption*. https://www.mondobirra.org/download/moderateconsuption.pdf

Burnley, I. H. (1974). International migration and metropolitan growth in Australia. In I. H. Burnley (Ed.), *Urbanization in Australia: The post-war experience* (Vol. 100–102). London: Cambridge University Press.

Crotty, M. (1998). *The foundations of social research*. Sydney: Allen & Unwin.

Crowther, E. (2013). *Eating culture: An anthropological guide to food*. Toronto: University of Toronto Press.

Daniel, M., Paquet, C., & McDermott, R. (2009). Obesity prevention in France: Yes, but how and why? *Public Health Nutrition, 12*(8), 2.

Dawson, T. (1597/1977). *The good huswifes jewell*. London: Walter J Johnson.

Economos, C. D., & Irish-Hauser, S. A. (2007). Community interventions: A brief overview and their application to the obesity epidemic. *The Journal of Law, Medicine & Ethics, 35*(1), 131–137.

Flynn, M. A. T., McNeil, D. A., Maloff, B., Mutasingwa, D., Wu, M., Ford, C., & Tough, S. C. (2006). Reducing obesity and related chronic disease risk in children and youth: A synthesis of evidence with 'best practice' recommendations. *Obesity Reviews, 7*, 7–66.

Forster, C., & McCaskill, M. (2007). The modern period: Managing metropolitan Adelaide. In A. Hutchings (Ed.), *With conscious purpose: A history of town planning in South Australia* (2nd ed., pp. 85–108a). Adelaide: Planning Institute of Australia (SA Division).

Glasse, H. (1747/1995). *The art of cookery made plain and easy*, by 'A Lady'. Totnes: Prospect Books.

Hansard. (2013). *House of Assembly, Estimates Committee B*, 26th June–2nd July 2013.

Hartwick, C. (2014). *Transferring an innovation in food and lifestyle education: Development of a French childhood obesity prevention program in Australia. A cultural comparison of childhood obesity prevention in France and Australia.* Unpublished PhD thesis, Université Paris Descartes Ecole doctorale SHS (ED180) CERLIS/Education et Formation and Flinders University School of Public Health, Adelaide.

Heuts, F., & Mol, A. (2013). What is a good tomato? A case of valuing in practice. *Valuation Studies, 1*(2), 125–146.

Heuzenroeder, A. (2006). European food meets Aboriginal food: To what extent did Aboriginal food cultures influence early German-speaking settlers in South Australia? *Limina, 12*, 30–39.

Hill, J. (2016). *On being a minister.* Adelaide: Wakefield Press.

Hordacre, A. L., Spoehr, J., Crossman, S., & Barbaro, B. (2013). *City of Playford socio-demographic, employment and education profile.* Adelaide: Australian Workplace Innovation and Social Research Centre.

Katan, M. (2009). Weight-loss diets for the prevention and treatment of obesity. *New England Journal of Medicine, 360*(9), 3.

Latour, B. (2000). When things strike back: A possible contribution of 'science studies' to the social sciences. *The British Journal of Sociology, 51*(1), 107–123.

Llewellyn-Smith, M. (2012). *Behind the scenes: The politics of planning Adelaide.* Adelaide: University of Adelaide Press.

Marsden, S. (Unknown). *Playford's metropolis.* www.sahistorians.org.au/175/bm.doc/playfords-metroplis-2.doc

McLachlan, R., Gilfillan, G., & Gordon, J. (2013). *Deep and persistent disadvantage in Australia. Productivity Commission report.* Canberra: Commonwealth of Australia.

Mendes, P. (2013). Compulsory income management: A critical examination of the emergence of conditional welfare in Australia. *Australian Social Work, 66*(4), 495–510.

Mol, A. (2012). Layers or versions? Human bodies and the love of bitterness. In B. Turner (Ed.), *The Routledge handbook of the body* (pp. 119–129). Oxford: Routledge.

OPAL. (2012). *OPAL guidebook*. SA Health, Government of South Australia.

Parkhurst-Ferguson, P. (2004). *Accounting for taste: The triumph of French cuisine*. Chicago: University of Chicago Press.

Parkhurst-Ferguson, P. (2014). *Word of mouth: What we talk about when we talk about food* (Vol. 50). Berkeley: University of California Press.

Peel, M. (1994a). A place made poor. *Arena Magazine* (Fitzroy, Victoria), *8*, 36–39.

Peel, M. (1994b). Making a place: Women in the workers' city. *Australian Historical Studies, 26*, 102, p. 2 (fn. 1).

Peel, M. (1995a). *Good times, hard times: The past and the future in Elizabeth*. Carlton: University of Melbourne.

Peel, M. (1995b). The rise and fall of social mix in an Australian new town. *Journal of Urban History, 22*(1), 108–140.

Peterson, K. E., & Fox, M. K. (2007). Addressing the epidemic of childhood obesity through school-based interventions: What has been done and where do we go from here? *The Journal of Law, Medicine & Ethics, 35*(1), 113–130.

Pisoni, D. (2008a, December 15). School weigh-in. *Today Tonight*. https://www.todaytonightadelaide.com.au/stories/school-weigh-in

Pisoni, D. (2008b). ABC news report. Retrieved from http://www.abc.net.au/news/2008-07-02/minister-knew-of-fast-food-link-to-nutrition/2491130

Playford Community Newsletter. (2012). *Spring into health with OPAL – City of Playford*. https://www.playford.sa.gov.au/webdata/resources/files/NIU%20low%20res%20for%20web_FINAL%2018.9.12.pdf. Accessed 20 May.

Poulain, J. P. (2002). The contemporary diet in France: 'De-structuration' or from commensalism to 'vagabond feeding'. *Appetite, 39*(1), 43–55.

Romon, M., Lommez, A., Tafflet, M., et al. (2009). Downward trends in the prevalence of childhood overweight in the setting of 12-year school- and community-based programmes. *Public Health Nutrition, 12*(10), 1735–1742.

Saberi, H., & Davidson, A. (2009). *Trifle*. Devon: Prospect Books.

Sanabria, E. (2015). Sensorial pedagogies, hungry fat cells and the limits of nutritional health education. *BioSocieties, 10*(2), 125–142.

Santich, B. (2011). Nineteenth-century experimentation and the role of Indigenous foods in Australian food culture. *Australian Humanities Review, 51*, 65–78.

Santich, B. (2012). *Bold palates: Australia's gastronomic heritage*. Adelaide: Wakefield Press.

Sato, K. (2013). Genetically modified food in France: Symbolic transformation and the policy paradigm shift. *Theory and Society, 42*(5), 477–507.

Shannon, P. (1995, September 6). The unfinished story of Elizabeth. *Green Left Weekly*, Issue 201. Retrieved from https://www.greenleft.org.au/content/unfinished-story-elizabeth

Summerbell, C. D., Douthwaite, W., Whittaker, V. J., Ells, L. J., Hillier, F. C., Smith, S., & Macdonald, I. A. R. (2009). The association between diet and physical activity and subsequent excess weight gain and obesity assessed at 5 years of age or older: A systematic review of the epidemiological evidence. *International Journal of Obesity, 33*(Supplement 3), S1–S92.

Swinburn, B., & de Silva-Sanigorski, A. (2010). Where to from here for preventing childhood obesity: An international perspective. *Obesity, 18*(Supplement 1), S4–S7.

Symons, M. (2007). *One continuous picnic: A gastronomic history of Australia*. Carlton: Melbourne University Press.

The Barossa Cookery book: 1000 selected recipes. (1932). Tanunda: Tanunda Institute Committee.

Townend, L. (2015). *Targeting healthy weight? How the ideologies and discourses underpinning the policies addressing South Australia's Healthy Weight Target (2007) affect health equity*. Unpublished PhD thesis, Southgate Institute for Society, Health and Equity, Flinders University of South Australia.

Uniting Communities and Community Centres. (2013). *An affordable place to live*. Adelaide: Government of South Australia.

van der Kleij, M. R., Crone, M., Reis, R., & Paulussen, T. (2016). Unravelling the factors decisive to the implementation of EPODE-derived community approaches targeting childhood obesity: A longitudinal, multiple case study. *International Journal of Behavioral Nutrition and Physical Activity, 13*(1), 98.

Venn, D., Banwell, C., & Dixon, J. (2017). Australia's evolving food practices: A risky mix of continuity and change. *Public Health Nutrition, 20*(14), 2549–2558.

Walker, R. B., & Roberts, D. C. K. (1988). Colonial food habits 1788–1900. In *Food habits in Australia. Proceedings of the first Deakin/Sydney Universities symposium on Australian nutrition* (pp. 40–59). Melbourne: Rene Gordon.

Warin, M. (2010). *Abject relations: Everyday worlds of anorexia*. New Brunswick: Rutgers University Press.

Warin, M., Turner, K., Moore, V., & Davies, M. (2008). Bodies, mothers and identities: Rethinking obesity and the BMI. *Sociology of Health & Illness, 30*(1), 97–111.

Warin, M., Zivkovic, T., Moore, V., Ward, P. R., & Jones, M. (2015). Short horizons and obesity futures: Disjunctures between public health interventions and everyday temporalities. *Social Science & Medicine, 128*, 309–315.

Warin, M., Zivkovic, T., Moore, V., & Ward, P. (2017). Moral fiber: Breakfast as a symbol of a 'good start' in an Australian obesity intervention. *Medical Anthropology: Cross-Cultural Studies in Health and Illness, 36*(3), 217–230.

Westley, H. (2007). Thin living. *British Medical Journal, 335*(7632), 1236–1237.

CHAPTER 4

Romantic Complexity and the Slippery Slope to Lifestyle Drift

There is a common belief in popular discourse that people are fat because they don't have the time to cook healthy meals, don't have the skills or know how to cook, or lack nutritional knowledge. For people living in circumstances of disadvantage, it is lack of skills and knowledge that is the accusation most frequently leveled at them. There is a wealth of scholarship that critiques the blaming of individuals for obesity (Evans et al. 2008; Gard and Wright 2005; Mayes 2016; Monaghan et al. 2013; Warin et al. 2015; Yates-Doerr 2015), and strong evidence that individual approaches have limited effectiveness (Baum 2011; Baum and Fisher 2014; Cohn 2014; Ulijaszek and McLennan 2016; Warin 2018). Despite this, individual responsibility remains the default position, and it is rare to hear public discussion or debate about social determinants of health, like poverty or unemployment in Australian obesity interventions and policy. Even when social determinants are mentioned, the focus always comes back to lifestyles and individual behaviors, which are presented as deficient and problematic. The international focus on "nudging" and social marketing in obesity campaigns speaks directly to this focus on individual behaviors, aimed *not* at the food industry, regulations, or alleviating poverty, but at the choices a person makes around food items or physical activity, or encouraging individuals to read and interpret food labels (c.f. Scrinis and Parker 2016).

The power of personal responsibility was evident in this headline of the state-based newspaper *The Advertiser* during our fieldwork: "Poverty no excuse for fat kids" (Bita 2013). The journalist cited research from a

M. Warin, T. Zivkovic, *Fatness, Obesity, and Disadvantage in the Australian Suburbs*,
https://doi.org/10.1007/978-3-030-01009-6_4

reputable Australian institute, which found that "[k]ids from poor families are three times more likely than the wealthiest kids to grow up obese." This journalist asks why:

> *A popular explanation from health professionals and academics is that disadvantaged families just can't afford to buy fresh, nutritious food. What tripe! A bunch of vitamin packed bananas costs less than a packet of fatty, salty chips or a cargo-charged ice-cream or chocolate bar … don't blame a lack of money for unhealthy eating.*

The implicit messages here draw upon well-worn tropes associated with obesity—laziness and ignorance. People who are obese and live in disadvantaged circumstances are constructed as "non-knowers" (Farrell et al. 2016, p. 6), not knowing which food is "good" (meaning nutritious) to eat, or how to shop for "the right foods." This style of thinking was evident in Farrell's research, where she examined class-based public perceptions about the use of preventive obesity measures in Australia. When people living in affluent areas of a major Australian city were asked about the "obesity problem," they immediately pointed to people in lower socioeconomic circumstances, rather than reflecting on their own body sizes. In supporting their opinions, they positioned themselves as "knowers," who know what to eat, how much to eat, and the right things to eat. Others, constructed as "epistemically disadvantaged" (Tuana 2006), ignorant of basic facts about nutrition, were seen to be in need of government information and education to "help them get over their own ignorance about things" (Farrell et al. 2016, p. 5). This participant from Farrell's study exemplifies this mantra:

> *Maybe they weren't taught to cook, they don't have those skills, so they accept crap food. They'll eat crap. I mean, personally, I wouldn't eat bad food, I just, I would go hungry [rather] than eat shit, but a lot people, you know, will eat that stuff and then suffer the consequences.* (Farrell et al. 2016, p. 4)

Moreover, this ignorance was seen to extend to inaccurate perceptions about the affordability of fresh food, as Scarlette from Obesity Prevention and Lifestyle (OPAL) summarized: "There's a perception that junk food is cheaper than fresh food." One suggested way to fix this problem was to educate those on low incomes about where to access healthy foods, on the assumption they wouldn't know where to find cheaper, healthy options.

Despite research undertaken directly in this geographical location that demonstrates the relative unaffordability of healthy foods (Ward et al. 2013), there was no attention drawn to "genuinely prohibitive cost barriers," poor access to healthy food outlets, or the difficulties of keeping perishable food fresh (ibid.). Another belief is that [disadvantaged] people knew what was deemed to be "good" and "bad" food but they willfully chose to eat foods which tasted nicer (Farrell et al. 2016; Zivkovic et al. 2015).

This not-knowing, or "information deficit model," is now dominant in public health interventions (Kowal 2015; Mayes and Thompson 2015; Warin 2018; Yates-Doerr 2015), where essentially it is thought that people need up-skilling in nutritional knowledge and cooking skills. In his elaborations of how we come to "know" things, Ingold (2013) critiques this "prepackaged" kind of information, arguing that it is authoritative knowledge that takes for granted the premise on which it is based. In this education model it is anticipated that social change will naturally occur once the community takes up new healthy behaviors. We found that some people in the community also thought this was the best approach to addressing obesity, like this shopper at a local supermarket:

> *People who are on benefits, welfare recipients, many of them complain that they don't have enough money but if you come in here on payday and you look in their trolleys it is full of pizzas and Coke® and chips and not real food. Many of them just do not know how to cook, no one has ever taught them so they don't know, and they don't know how to spend their money to buy food that is good and healthy for their families. So I think that some of their welfare money should be given to them in food vouchers to buy healthy food like fruit and veg and stuff to make a meal, and they should also have to do cooking classes. I mean I cook because my mum always cooked and she showed me. So then when I had kids I cooked and then taught them and now they both cook, but lots of people here do not know how; their mothers did not know how. It is generational. Someone needs to teach them.*

This chapter examines the ideological underpinnings of the OPAL program, focusing on how the deficit model of knowledge was at the heart of the social marketing and delivery of education, particularly around nutrition. Despite the rhetoric of a socioecological approach to obesity, the first aim of the OPAL program was directed to individual behaviors, looking to increase "healthy eating through reducing energy-dense nutrient-poor food consumption and increasing nutritious food consumption" in the community. We argue that three key factors were at play in implementing this aim: the construction of the community as "not-knowing" and in need of educational up-skilling; the "black-boxing" of nutritional discourse (Sanabria 2016; Scrinis 2013; Yates-Doerr 2012, 2015); and the construction of obesity as a form of romantic complexity (Kwa 2002; Ulijaszek 2015, 2017). Implicit in this model was the neoliberal assumption that OPAL would, as one manager stated, "mobilize responsibility," enabling individuals to take responsibility for their nutritional intake and make behavioral changes to improve their eating habits. As we demonstrate, this enabled the socioecological approach to slide into a focus on lifestyle behaviors—what Carey et al. (2017) refer to as the "lifestyle drift."

Guidebooks, Roadmaps, and "the Bible": Improving Health Literacy

What is eating? What is healthy eating? What is unhealthy eating? These were key questions in our ethnographic project: we were interested in how people ate, and daily activities that are performed around such practices. Such simple and taken-for-granted questions give rise to many different interpretations. As anthropologists we came with an understanding of food and eating as deeply embedded in tacit sociocultural practices, and contingent on the many social relationships, practices, memories, tastes, circumstances, and a wide range of social determinants (gender, race, and ethnicity, employment, housing, age) that influence and impact on everyday lives. We recognized that public health, health promotion, and nutrition were similarly shaped by certain knowledges and values (with a range of understandings), and that these were also deeply ingrained in epistemological framings. We were also highly trained in Bourdieurian and Foucauldian theories, aware of the "tastes" of differing classes, the power of "hegemonic nutrition" (Hayes-Conroy and Hayes-Conroy 2013, pp. 1–2), and the working of biopower through standardization, normalization, and disciplining of bodies. We were also aware that different versions of health, bodies, and eating could be enacted depending on particular circumstances, and that bodies were not singular or universal functioning units (c.f. Mol 2012a).

As discussed in Chap. 2, the OPAL project (in the scientific committee meetings and local teams) did not need to interrogate the concept of healthy eating. There was no substantive debate over the nature of the problem of obesity in our fieldwork location, as "poor eating" had already been identified, and linked explicitly to obesity and disadvantage. Health data were used as evidence for the need for intervention. For example, Poppy (an OPAL manager) used survey data to characterize the community as unhealthy and at heightened risk of lifestyle diseases. With the data in hand, she compared the community with standard benchmarks: "Do people do the recommended amount of physical activity?—No." "They do drink a lot of sweetened drinks." "They will end up developing obesity-related chronic conditions." Coupled with a fieldwork location that did have high numbers of fast food outlets when compared with other suburbs in the city, and small, local supermarkets that had limited choices in terms of food options, Playford was an ideal place to invest in behavioral change. OPAL workers wanted the community to thrive and to become "a place more than [just] sausages, mince, and smokes" (Max, OPAL manager).

Before the OPAL program was launched in any community, a "roadmap" pack was given to OPAL teams by local councils, to advertise to people that "OPAL has come to town." Derived from the EPODE advice to French communities, the pack outlined the steps required to successfully implement the program, and that key outcomes would be reported. Also included was a suite of standardized resources; for example: OPAL PowerPoint presentations, "Introducing OPAL" brochures, sample letters to stakeholders, "core corporate communication tools," and specific instructions on how to deal with the media. During the course of the program, each new theme would be also accompanied by another roadmap, articulating that theme's key strategies and desired outcomes. For the *Screen Time* theme, for example, the importance of active play and physical activity was highlighted by means of the accompanying tools and merchandise (posters, hopscotch kits, Frisbees, skipping ropes) all of which could be distributed in the community to support the theme.

When a new council area joined the OPAL program, they were supplied with a lengthy OPAL guidebook of 125 pages. On several occasions it was reiterated to us that the guidebook was for stakeholders only, and not intended for the general community. Known by OPAL staff as "the Bible," this was intended to be used as a reference tool to help staff understand the background, structure, and governance of the program. Following a classic Foucauldian approach, the guidebook provided evidence as to why obesity was a problem (illustrated with national and state-based graphs and statistics), and reiterated the French story to establish legitimacy for the uptake of OPAL. Early on in the guide, it was stated that Stage 1 of EPODE started with the delivery of a five-year "educating through information" program. Just as preschoolers and primary school children in Fleurbaix and Laventie were taught a nutritional information program that would be delivered by their teachers, this was similarly a major tenet of the OPAL program.

In the OPAL guidebook, the authors identified that "nutrition and health prevention are areas in which many preconceived ideas and personal beliefs are expressed." It wasn't clear what these ideas were, but the implication was that "personal beliefs" stood in contrast to the facts of nutrition and needed to be changed. One main strategy in changing these preconceived ideas was to use social marketing to change behaviors. As in the EPODE context, the aim of social marketing was to bring about "sustained changes in social norms through an environment that stimulates the adoption of health-promoting behaviors." Again, it wasn't clear what these "social norms" that needed changing were. While the guidebook was careful not to overtly blame individuals for poor eating habits, the implicit and underlying discourse suggests that target communities did not exhibit good health behaviors. Max (an OPAL manager) supported this assumption in an interview, when he stated: "We need to change unhealthy behavior to a healthy behavior."

This implicit understanding underpinned the OPAL program. Communities were specifically selected to participate if they had high levels of overweight and obesity and were identified as disadvantaged based on statistical data on low socioeconomic status derived from Australia's national census figures. The city of Palmerston in the Northern Territory was also part of OPAL, included so as to "target the Indigenous population" (and was there rebranded as Childhood Obesity Prevention and Lifestyle [COPAL]).

Class, race, and obesity were thus intimately linked, and corrective behavioral messages planned via a strong social marketing program. One of OPAL's "behavioral change specialists" explained to us that new "social marketing themes were originally put forward every 6 months, but in the second year this was extended to every 12 months." Themes were presented in posters, brochures, community education sessions, and fact sheets, and via a range of branded products (e.g. plastic bowls for eating breakfast cereal, plastic water bottles, lunch box tags). The posters and brochures were designed to "raise awareness" and "provide basic key messages" (OPAL guidebook, p. 38) (Fig. 4.1).

Whether it was physical activity, screen time, or healthy eating, the message was clear that children and families were spending too much time in

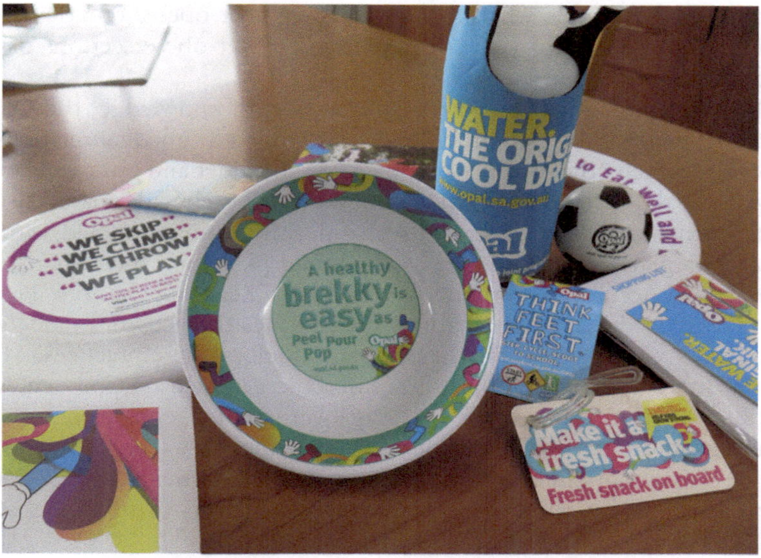

Fig. 4.1 Some of the OPAL social marketing products. (Photo from Authors)

front of screens, drinking too many soft drinks, eating the wrong types of foods, and not playing outdoors. Children's bodies were conceived as engines, taking in too much fuel and putting out too little energy, drawing on industrial metaphors of metabolism as combustion (Landecker 2011). As with the "eat less and exercise more" mantra, the "less" of one thing and "more" of another characterized families as not knowing the "basic facts" about healthy eating and physical activity (OPAL guidebook, p. 101).

Interviews with some staff intimately involved with the OPAL program reiterated this lack of knowledge. As well as identifying the costs and time required to "being active and eating well," one OPAL worker stated: "I think it's quite clear that they [families in Playford] don't have the underpinning education, or at least literacy, to be able to navigate the world that they find themselves in to enhance their health and well-being." This assumption was well-intended and situated within a benevolent public health framework looking to improve people's lives, but it positioned people as ignorant in terms of knowing what and how to eat. We always wondered if this sort of deficit knowledge statement would similarly be directed at middle-class people who are also overweight or obese. What explanations would be put forward for well-educated yet obese sections of the population?

In this conventional and hierarchical model of knowledge, the OPAL staff and people in the community are positioned in unequal relations of power, in which "the sender is perceived as the holder and giver of 'knowledge' and the receiver as without 'knowledge'" (Schneidermann 2018). With such morality-laden discourses of healthy eating, coupled with an explicit target on disadvantage, the program planners expect that social change will occur as a community adopts new healthy behaviors. People simply need education about nutrition and healthy activities, and once they know what is good for them, they will adopt these practices. Many commentators have noted the power imbalances in such an approach, with Lupton suggesting incisively that "[g]overnment agencies engaged in health promotion, and the commercial companies they consult to assist in their efforts, continue to rely on simplistic, paternalistic, and reductionist approaches to educating the public and attempting to instill behavior change" (Lupton 2014, p. 45).

"A Patron Saint for OPAL"

Coveney has carefully investigated the ways in which nutrition science is more than a reductionist science, arguing that it acts more broadly (and productively) as a template of historical and contemporary moral ordering, in which judgments about ourselves and others are encoded in science and religious discourses (Coveney 2006, p. xiii). Using Foucault's work on governmentality, Coveney discusses how knowledge of food can be understood as a "discipline" in two senses: first as field of scientific endeavor, and second as a form of moral correction (1999, p. x, see also Evans et al. 2008). In explicating his arguments, Coveney traces the historical antecedents of Western breakfast cereals, demonstrating the moral and spiritual values inscribed in their making, and how these values are deeply engrained in virtues of "goodness" and "peristaltic governance" (Warin et al. 2017).

OPAL was invested in the promotion of breakfast as a meal, and certain breakfast cereals. The story that has particular relevance to our focus starts in the early years of the twentieth century at a Michigan-based Seventh Day Adventist–run health resort, The Battle Creek Sanitarium. It was here that Adventists developed new food in accordance with the diet recommended by the church, experimenting with a number of different grains. The nutritional philosophy of the Adventists emphasized eating foods in their most simple and natural form, the way that "God provided for our use" (White 1905/2015, p. 313). Foods that imparted flavor and pleasure (such as meat from pigs, alcohol, spices, or sweet foods) were carnal pleasures to be especially avoided because of their power to constipate and contaminate the body, stimulating animal passions and leading to sins of the flesh—principally masturbation (Warin et al. 2017). Wealthy Americans flocked to "the San" to engage in strict dietary and hygienic practices, in a quest for spiritual and social purity. In promoting the health-enhancing effects of dieting and purging practices (such as enemas), the Sanitorium changed its name to the Sanitarium. Interestingly, the Adventists' focus on fiber (roughage) here occurred well before mainstream medicine's recognition of its benefits for bowel health in the 1950s (Kritchevsky 1988).

Cornflakes® were developed by Dr. John Harvey Kellogg, then superintendent of the Sanitarium, when he serendipitously created flakes from cooked grain that had unintentionally gone stale. A patent on the process was acquired, cornflakes became hugely popular, and rival breakfast cereal manufacturers soon opened in the Battle Creek area. This competition fueled Will Keith Kellogg's (Dr. Kellogg's brother) desire to use his entrepreneurial skills to market the new food for mass consumption. Will bought the rights from his brother and set up the Kellogg Toasted Corn Flake Company, discarding the health angle and adding sugar for palatability (Wilson 2014).[1] At around the same time, a young Australian Adventist minister, who had been a patient at the Sanitarium, returned to Melbourne and started the Sanitarium Health Food Agency, which shredded compressed wheat into what would become Weet-Bix®. Marketed as a "health biscuit," Weet-Bix® is presented as the breakfast of historical and current sporting champions and heroes: soldiers on the front line in World War I (WWI) were said to eat it, and it is the Australian cricket team's official cereal. There is thus a clear association with Australian identity, extending from nationalist pride to healthy, young Australian children. As the company's advertising slogan proclaims, "Aussie kids," after all, "are Weet-Bix® kids" (Warin et al. 2017).

The transformative power of food to "uplift" and "save" people was noticed by participants in the field—both stakeholders and members of the community. At a stakeholder consultation workshop in Playford, prior to the launch of OPAL in 2009, a Playford councilor told us that it was good that OPAL was focusing on children, and not "worrying about the adults—it's too late, they're a lost cause." Children are the ones to be "saved," as they are a convenient (and captive) population for regulation and intervention (Coveney 2008; Dehghan et al. 2005; Zivkovic et al. 2010), and they represent future generations of obese adults, and bodily sites to target to prevent such medical and socioeconomic disaster (Wang and Dietz 2002). The saving of children was to be accomplished by OPAL workers, who used the OPAL "Bible" and identified themselves to children as role models. As one OPAL manager from a regional council area put it, "[w]e must walk the walk and practice what we preach."

OPAL workers were described by some participants as "incredibly fit," "healthy," middle-class health professionals who "spread messages." In this scenario the local mayor was presented as a "sort of patron saint for OPAL," a male figure of imposing girth who often appeared in public in his flowing, red, velvet-edged, and faux fur–trimmed mayoral robes, complete with gold medallion. This representation of OPAL as a quasi-religious movement conforms to traditional public health models of behavioral change that try to present information and provide incentives so individuals can make "better choices for themselves" (Shove et al. 2012, p. 144).

Jamie Oliver's crusade, the *Ministry of Food*, is perhaps the best exemplar of this transformative approach and governing crusade. Oliver was labeled by the residents of the northern English town of Rotherham as a "messiah," and his apprentices as "apostles." Mick the miner "had an epiphany" after making a dish, when he discovered that "men really could cook" (Warin 2011). However, after their outrage at the limited and selective way in which Oliver represented Rotherham to the world, some locals wanted to "nail [Jamie] to a cross." And the author of the *Jamie Go Home* blog cynically commented: "Thank goodness a missionary came to show us posh ham and asparagus" (https://jamiegohome.wordpress.com/about/). Foucault would appreciate this analogy, as he believed that medical and religious regimes are both aesthetic disciplines focused on the government of the body.

"Knowledge Based on Science": Focusing on Nutrition

The OPAL manager at our field site, Poppy, was a dietician, and there were numerous times when we accidentally referred to her as a nutritionist, which led to swift correction. We became aware of the hierarchy of expert status that such categorizations entail, acknowledging the higher level of qualification as a form of symbolic capital. In Australia, all dietitians and nutritionists are educated through tertiary institutions, and can provide evidence-based advice on nutrition services. All dietitians are nutritionists, but they have taken additional training in clinical nutrition and individual dietary counseling, and are accredited according to industry standards (e.g. Dietary Association of Australia). The backgrounds of most OPAL staff were in nutrition and dietetics, social marketing, sports science, and exercise physiology, with one educated in the social sciences. Notably, most of the OPAL staff were young women.

Poppy was described by other stakeholders as "staunch" in her approach to food and eating, in that she judged foods by their nutritional content and followed a strict discourse of healthism. Crawford (1980) coined the term "healthism" to critique a particular emphasis on a new health consciousness that divided human activity into "approved and disapproved, healthy and unhealthy, prescribed and proscribed, responsible and irresponsible" (Skrabanek 1994, cited in Mayes 2016, p. 2). While there are various political slants on healthism (for an overview, see Mayes 2016, p. 62), it is no longer a top-down approach of state interventions, but part and parcel of neoliberal ideals that citizens are expected to engage in choices that empower them to be healthy. Making the right, educated choices is an exemplar of Foucault's (1990) concept of biopower and governmentality, demonstrating the political tactics that are entailed in encouraging individuals to make healthy choices that improve not only their health, but the health of the population.

In this context, food was directly related to health and ill-health, and circumscribed with the values of good nutrition, determined by the correct caloric intake, balance of carbohydrates, proteins, and fats, and limiting "sometimes foods." It wasn't surprising that this view was concomitant with the federal Australian Government's "Australian Guide to Healthy Eating," a poster showing a pie chart divided into the five (nutritious) food groups. This was a ubiquitous image at our field sites (appearing at community education sessions and food banks), positioned as the authoritative information from "the best available scientific evidence" about what types of foods we should be eating, and in what quantities. As a piece of key and often initially presented information, the Guide to Healthy Eating was presented as normative and accumulated knowledge, but it made no allusion to the sociality of eating or the myriad complexities and decisions that come with accessing food (Warin et al. 2015; Warin 2018) (Fig. 4.2).

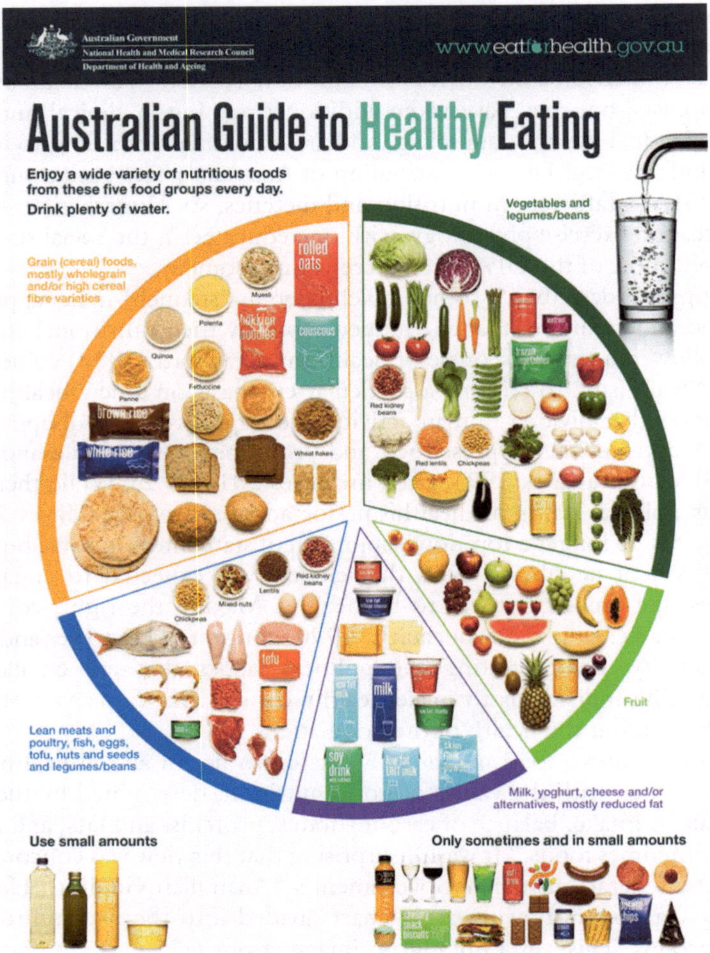

Fig. 4.2 Australian Government's *Australian Guide to Healthy Eating*. (Source: https://tinyurl.com/yby2w29z)

At community education sessions the chart enabled OPAL workers to teach participants about nutrients, vitamins, minerals, and portion sizes. "What's a superfood?" asked Scarlette at a meeting of Community Foodies (for detailed explanation on Community Foodies, see page 111). A woman calls out "broccoli." "Yes, that's right, broccoli is a superfood. It's packed with vitamins and minerals. Broccoli even has more vitamin C than oranges." The next week Scarlette asks: "What are whole foods?" No one answers so she continues: "These are the foods that are shown here [on the Australian Guide to Healthy Eating]. These foods are low in saturated fats, sugar, and salt, all of which abound in processed, packaged foods that put pressure on our organs to function. In contrast, *these* foods are good for memory, concentration, and general brain function."

What was interesting about these sessions was that no participants spoke about food as nutrients in their everyday conversations. They didn't talk about foods as high in protein, or how many vitamins or minerals certain foods contained. They didn't talk about "whole foods" or "superfoods" in their everyday worlds. There was some talk of the amount of sugar in soft drinks (and the "Guess the Sugar" game was a favorite OPAL teaching resource and often on display), but generally this nutrient typology description of food was remarkably absent in fieldwork encounters.

What community people did talk about was how illness (such as diabetes, cancer, or depression) influenced their choice and enjoyment of foods. Jude, for example, who had multiple health problems (cancer, diabetes, and lupus) needed to be careful with all her food and couldn't eat some fresh foods (like capsicum) as they disagreed with her stomach. As a qualified Community Foodie she had been asked to give talks to all the people who underwent gastric bypass surgery at the local public hospital, as they could only access a free consultation with a nutritionist twice a year, and the nurses reported that many people post-surgery were eating packets of chips. Many other participants talked about dealing with chronic mental health issues, including depression and anxiety, and the ways in which this impacted on their bodies. Thirty-six-year-old Philippa explained that "when people are struggling with their lives they tend to look for something else to make things better … and food, alcohol, drugs seem to be the things of choice." Coping with postnatal depression and a partner in jail, she escaped the realities of life with "ice, meth and speed," becoming so skinny that you could see her heart beating through her ribs: "I had people telling that I was getting too skinny so I was like, 'I'll fix this.' Cake and cream, cake and cream every day—I was just smashing out the cake and cream and then I just exploded back up to a size 12 to a 14 and I was like, 'I'm too fat again.'"

Food, in the OPAL context, was reduced to what staff called "basic nutrition"; simplified messages about different components, decontextualized from everyday realities of eating that are tempered by precariousness as well as the sharing and enjoyment of foods. A clear example involved the social marketing of the breakfast theme. Social marketing brochures for the "healthy brekky" theme provided a step-by-step guide to help people make "good choices" in selecting a healthy breakfast. There were three steps to remember:

Step 1: Consider the nutrition information panel.
Step 2: Consider the ingredient list.
Step 3: Consider the nutritional claims on cereal boxes.

These steps included assessing the energy, fat, protein, carbohydrate, sugar, sodium, and dietary fiber of a product, based on the first three or four ingredients of each product, and "reading carefully" the nutrition and health claims of a product.

While label-reading was core practice in OPAL education sessions and Foodies training, people did not shop like this in the local food banks. They checked some labels—especially price tags and expiry dates on the "specials" table—but not nutritional labeling. In the food bank people spoke about adding sugar to breakfast cereals (and sugar was one of the biggest purchases), but never checking the quantity of sugar already in the product.

Even if nutrition labels are looked at, it might not be with the intention of rejecting that item. One day in the food bank a local worker, Katie, commented on the grapefruit drink she'd just finished. Holding out the empty bottle in front of her, she said: "Well, that was quite nice. I thought I'd better try it because we haven't had it before and the customers will ask what it's like. I quite like grapefruit." Tanya tells her that she prefers grapefruit if it's got some sugar in it to sweeten the sour taste. "Me too," Katie laughed. "Is there much sugar in the drink?" Tanya asked, assuming that the sugar content would be high. Katie read the back label and her mouth dropped: "This is 20% sugar—there is a lot of added sugar—the sodium content is high too. Oh dear, I should have just had water. … I could have had a chocolate bar instead," she sighed, as she walked to the back of the shop, empty bottle in hand.

Several food scholars have noted the reductionist tendencies of nutritional advice, referring to this as "nutritional black-boxing" (Yates-Doerr 2015, p. 56) or nutritional reductionism (Scrinis 2008, 2013). Scrinis has long argued that the nutrition industry, including nutrition scientists, dieticians, and public health authorities, has "come to dominate, to undermine, and to replace other ways of engaging with food and of contextualizing the relationship between food and the body" (2008, p. 39). He suggests that this is directly related to the food industry's marketing strategies, in which the abstract and neutral language of nutrients (rather than processing techniques) is used to obscure the profound influence of the food industry. Elevating nutrients as the primary relationship people have with food, both in terms of the quality of foods and their relationships to bodily health, is a form of nutritional reductionism. He suggests that

> *[t]he mandatory nutrient information panel on the back of packaged foods that details their nutrient composition is, in a sense, a product and a symbol of first-order reductionism, particularly when it appears more prominently than the ingredients list.* (Scrinis 2008, p. 41)

In her ethnographic work on obesity in Guatemala, Yates-Doerr argues: "Health is not a property that can be fixed within a food; [it exists] instead in the specificities of dietary practices, it is a process to be enacted, not an object to hold" (Yates-Doerr 2015, p. 307). This process is embedded in the phenomenological experiences of foods, and the many emotional registers (pleasure, disgust, remembering) and social relationships that eating entails. OPAL, however, used a public education model in which the science of healthy eating was seen as something separate from society. In this model, dieticians and nutritionists hold the expert knowledge and have to instruct and educate the public—and the public do not intervene in the process of knowledge transfer. This knowledge transmission model of education is already formed: "An induction into the rules and representations" (Ingold 2013, p. 1) of what constitutes healthy eating. This is also the school classroom model, where pupils' minds are filled with accumulated knowledge from the past, often from experts. In this understanding, knowledge is information. The assumption here is that if people are given this knowledge as information, they can follow through with a rational and logical mode of knowing: "[They can] attend to the communication, understand the information it contains, remember that information, believe it to be true, and integrate it with his or her existing knowledge" (Prentice 2015, p. 268; Warin 2018). Moreover, this approach operates on the assumption that if people are given information, then their eating behaviors will change regardless of any other priorities or stressors they are dealing with.

One of the most glaring examples of the inadequacy of the "science mode" of nutrition education occurred when local council workers delivered a nutrition training session with local Burundian families who had migrated from East Africa. About eight Burundian migrants came to the session at a community living skills center. The Burundian men sat in silence until more women arrived, young children attached to their backs with large brightly colored floral cloths, hugging them tightly. The Anglo volunteers running the session—Faith and Rose—began with the familiar image of the Australian Guide to Healthy Eating (AGHE), with an interpreter translating in Kirundi. An African man had already told us that the foods he buys from the Afghan, Chinese, and African shops were not classified in the table depicted on the poster, and we wondered how people might respond to the message.

The group is told that it's important to monitor their serving sizes, especially in terms of controlling their weight. When told that a serving of meat should fit in their hand, they all take out their hands and look at their palms and laugh—saying through the interpreter that they eat much larger portions of meat than what is being recommended. Tanya recalls a conversation circling in different fieldwork spaces about a Burundian woman who bought a dead goat from the central food markets in the city and brought it back on the bus. The goat was to be cooked for families to share, but people on the bus complained about the dead goat on public transport and the woman was fined. As there is no fine for carrying a dead goat on public transport, the woman was fined for jaywalking. Tanya smiled at this story, aware that portion size is not part of the Burundian practices of sharing meats.

Then they are told to choose meat with less fat on it or to trim the fat off. The interpreter translates again from a woman who shouts: "She is saying that it is the best part and that the really fatty part tastes so good when it is cooked under the grill." "We agree," says one of the educators, "but this is about what is good for us, not what we think tastes best. The fatty part of the meat will make you fat and it is bad for your heart too." This negation of the sensory pleasures of taste are common in dieting and nutrition advice, suggesting that people must "overrule the desires of [their] craving body" (Mol 2012b, p. 379) in the interests of weight loss, thus enacting a Cartesian distinction of a rational mind over an unruly body.

Romantic Complexity and the Socioecological Model

What stood out with the OPAL program (and no doubt captured political attention of those who brought the program to Australia) was its stated focus on addressing socioecological factors that contribute to obesity. In the OPAL materials provided to staff and stakeholders, and in public presentations, this socioecological approach was described in various ways—as a methodology, a theoretical methodology, and sometimes as an ecological system. The approach is summed up by OPAL staff in one of their publications:

> *The Ecological Systems approach brings to the foreground the dynamic interrelations of variables in the social environments* (Bronfenbrenner 1977). *Human physiology and behavior (i.e. genetics, energy balance, eating and nutritional habits, sleep and exercise regimens); levels of income and food purchasing patterns; the built environment that impacts spaces for play and exercise; food supply and access issues, are some of the contributing factors to obesity. Through applying the socio-ecological approach/model OPAL staff keep a sharp focus on both individual and environmental/structural changes, at the same time. OPAL's approach is holistic in the active recognition that it takes far more than the health sector to address the challenges of rising obesity rates* (Australian Bureau Statistics 2013; Obesity Australia 2014). *Many other sectors influence behaviors and social environments that have an impact on nutrition and physical activity. For example, through the data entered into the Single Platform more than 35 sectors/industries have been identified.* (OPAL Collective 2015, p. 4)

To demonstrate this holistic approach, the OPAL team developed a "logic model" to understand the complexity of obesity, and the relationships between various sectors. The logic model is described as "theoretically informed" (OPAL Collective 2015, p. 6) and "consistent with the typical logic model flow" (2015, p. 4) in its four parts: resources and inputs, activities and outputs, impacts, and outcomes (ibid.).

The social marketing arm is described as "at OPAL's core" (ibid.), drawing on "technical, rational, interdisciplinary evidence to formulate specific themes," which were implemented at all OPAL sites. The themes were devised by the OPAL Scientific Advisory Committee (comprised 16 South Australian academics with expertise mainly in endocrinology, marketing, economics, psychology, epidemiology, and nutrition) and included water, active play, healthy snacks, active travel, breakfast, and outdoor play. At one of the statewide OPAL training days held in Adelaide, the OPAL social marketing team described its activities as

> *the systematic application of marketing alongside other concepts and techniques, to achieve specific behavioral goals for social good … the person is at the center of all we do … the consumer is the focus, not the product. In the case of OPAL, the child is at the center. So although we may have to change the behavior of parents and change policy, it is the child who is at the center of health promotion and social marketing.*

While we heard many references to a "socioecological model" and many staff firmly believed in this approach, this was superficial and there was little evidence that this was embedded into the program itself. There is a wealth of academic literature on social determinants of health, but this factor seemed to be completely absent from OPAL publications (which was surprising) or social marketing. When we interviewed Max (an OPAL manager), he mentioned the public health figure who has led the social determinants and health inequity campaign internationally, Professor Michael Marmot, and readily acknowledged the influence of social connectedness, employment, and education on life chances. "We're grounded in that," he said, "and from a social determinants perspective we recognize simply eating well and being active is not enough … but our focus is really about trying to increase levels of physical activity amongst a family and [to look at] the quality of food that they are consuming." In using the rhetoric of a socioecological model, OPAL might think it is changing the narrative, but it consistently reverts to a simple and linear model.

What prevents OPAL from broadening its scope to incorporate social determinants of health is the dominance of a causal narrative. In examining the puzzle of why the wealth of evidence and scholarship on the impact of social determinants of health has not had more impact on policy and practice, Kelly and Russo (2018) suggest that we rely too much on simple, causal narratives in public health. They argue that once risks are identified (overeating or not eating the right kinds of food, not taking enough exercise), they

> *are attributed to the consequences of people's behaviors and lifestyles or their inability to make healthy choices. Therefore, in order to reduce exposure to these risks, interventions to change behaviors and lifestyles are required. In other words, once a plausible account of the etiology of the disease is established (the risky behavior), it is assumed that acting on the same mechanisms (the behavior) will reduce the burden of disease.* (Kelly and Russo 2018, p. 2)

Yet it is not always the case that the "mechanisms of etiology of disease are the same as the mechanisms to prevent disease" (ibid.). In Max's account, OPAL avoided the complexity of people's everyday behaviors and practices and defaulted to an easier and simpler model of aiming to reduce people's food intake and increase their physical activity.

What was also strikingly absent in the OPAL program logic model was any critique of multinational food corporations, industry forces, food production, or any attention to class, gender, ethnicity, Indigenous status, or poverty. A health worker in the community spoke to us about this gap:

> *Before [OPAL] we used to take poverty seriously, community programs were oriented towards addressing real issues that were identified by community members themselves but now the funding of programs are about health issues that impact on government money only, and not the range of social factors that shape those health problem[s] ... it comes back to the individual, they are blamed for their problem [obesity] and not all the other factors that are involve[d] ... no-one in SA Health is pointing the finger at McDonalds®, it's the fault of the people living here, not the fault of modern capitalism. (Ruth)*

Equity is a "principle" of OPAL, but this is mainly discussed in relation to the desire not to stigmatize community members who are obese, and to address issues of affordability and access. The latter was addressed through what Poppy described as "environmental responsibility," creating places that are easier and safer to use (bike paths, walking trails) and working with a local supermarket manager to change the availability of unhealthy meats (from bacon, mince, and sausages to leaner meats like chicken). These are positive initiatives but, in not attending to corporate and government responsibility, the OPAL logic model is a functionalist model that aims to address complexity through holism, integrating multiple sites of intervention (the environment and the individual) to reach a final outcome based on the individual measurement of "healthy weight."

These types of socioecological models are common in health presentations concerning obesity, and as Sanabria notes, are "the classic set of categories that appear in the literature on health promotion" (2016, p. 143). These hierarchical categories place the individual as a key entity either at the bottom or in the center of the model, enveloped by other circles which are seen to shape behavior, such as the interpersonal organizational community and, at the broadest level, the societal/policy influences. This holistic model (or whole-systems model) is what some authors refer to as "romantic complexity" (Kwa 2002; Sanabria 2016; Ulijaszek 2015) as it is founded on the idea of "hierarchical levels of organization integrated into a functional whole, [aiming] to provide a coherent model of complex systems by mapping the relationships between constitutive elements" (Sanabria 2016, p. 146).

The effect of mapping obesity in this romantic framing, as Ulijaszek argues, is to make visible and knowable all the different components of obesity. Placing the individual at the center of such knowing, with arrows that flow to the other levels of influence, make it appear that all these components are "joined up" and lifestyles can be changed just through attention to healthy eating and physical activity. There is no room for the dynamics of power—of contestation, resistance, protest, contradiction, or the messiness of lives—let alone other epistemological framings or the political and economic influences of industry, trade, or agriculture lobbies. Such a model would not be romantic, but spring from a baroque sensibility, presenting complexity as endless and impossible to know fully (Law 2004 cited in Sanabria 148; Ulijaszek 2015), and with no assumptions of coherence. But baroque complexity cannot be managed by bureaucracies, reduced to an evidence base, or measured as a body mass index (BMI) output.

At one OPAL state training day when all the OPAL workers across the state traveled to Adelaide, a manager from a different council area noted the tension in the OPAL logic between the socioecological approach and the sharp focus on changing individual behavior through social marketing. Following a presentation from two social marketers he raised a key question:

> *Social marketing? So it's an individual approach. Maybe what needs to change is more about the policy, the decision makers, the policy makers—and so maybe they should be at the center rather than the individual so that we don't just get tied into individual responsibility … in an era where we live with self-responsibility and people governing themselves and then being measured—I mean, we've got to put the checks in.* (Martin, OPAL manager)

Martin was a lone voice of criticism, and his comments were swept aside in the nodding of the presenters, who didn't appear to follow the critique he was making or the contradiction that he was pointing out. They assumed he was complimenting the socioecological approach and that he agreed with the prevailing view that OPAL was innovative.

Martin's question points to the reductionist effects of romantic modeling. Following the arrows of the logic model, complexity is reduced to a focus on healthy eating and physical activity behaviors, leading ultimately to healthy weight of individuals. A similar romantic framing occurred in the UK's Foresight Obesity Systems Map (Ulijaszek 2015), where energy balance (again, between food and physical activity) was placed at the center of the model, excluding the development of solutions directly involving the many vested interests that make profits from activities that promote obesity, either directly or indirectly (Guthman 2011; Ulijaszek 2015, p. 216).

This reductionist process of romantic complexity leads to "lifestyle drift"—where community-based health programs start off with a broad social determinants (upstream) approach in their rhetoric of delivery, but then drift downstream to largely individual lifestyle factors (Baum 2011; Hunter et al. 2010). Australian commentators have noted how this is particularly the case in obesity initiatives, in which a community-level obesity initiative turns into a social marketing campaign encouraging individual physical activity, with a particular emphasis on the most disadvantaged groups (Lupton 2014). This was certainly the case with OPAL, where the council manager was responsible for "behavior change programs in the areas of physical activity and healthy eating." Although a social context might be acknowledged, the primacy of individuals and their choices is strongly maintained via the concept of health behavior (Cohn 2014, p. 159). In the next section, we examine how this OPAL logic model worked to circumvent knowledge, having lassoed the parameters via a cohesive framework that excluded the diversity of understandings about food, bodies, and eating held by community participants.

"You Can't Just Override People's Tastes, Can You?"

In our fieldwork we participated in educational training sessions led by OPAL workers for people in the community. One of these was with a group called Community Foodies, a South Australian nutrition program that operates across the state and trains local volunteers in healthy food choices. Volunteers who sign up for training undertake six sessions of training, and on completion are known as "Foodies" who can then work in their local community to help support others in making healthy eating choices. Trained Foodies are actively involved as peer educators in a wide variety of community settings, including childcare centers, aged care, community events, workplaces, and community centers. At the time of our project, the main aim of Community Foodies was to increase nutritional literacy in communities, especially among those most disadvantaged, including newly arrived families, Aboriginal and Torres Strait Islander families, those living with poor mental health, the elderly, and children living in poverty. In 2014, the State Government Department of Health (SA Health) appointed a church organization to lead and manage Community Foodies and, in a letter to all volunteers in this program, noted how the church agency has "a wealth of experience in working with vulnerable and disadvantaged communities."

Tanya participated in a Northern Community Foodies training session during the OPAL project, which was run in the home economics room at a local primary school. The room was set up with six ovens and three double sinks and a group of tables set out to resemble a standard teaching space (high tables with bar stools and lower tables with standard chairs). Despite being surrounded by cooking technologies, the sessions were focused on educating the participants, not on the practice of cooking.

For the sessions Tanya participated in, the 26 participants (25 women and 1 man) were a mixture of local people (including recently arrived migrants from Sudan and South Africa) and some from other areas of Adelaide who had traveled for over two hours to participate. OPAL was very respectful of programs that were already running in the community, and tried to link in with existing events rather than reinvent the wheel. Northern Community Foodies was already well established in the area and had four key messages that were very much in tune with the OPAL mantra: eat breakfast; eat more fruit and vegetables; drink more water; eat more whole foods. Rachel, the local facilitator, who usually ran the course, was a woman of average build in her fifties with graying hair and a somewhat gruff personality. She took a back seat while the two OPAL staff, Scarlette and Amelia, led the course. Both were employees of the State Government Department of Health and trained respectively in dietetics and human movement/health studies. They arrived first thing in the morning with armfuls of food (cheesy risotto balls, pumpkin soup, and jugs of water) prepared by a local community center that provides cheap meals for people in need, and props (bottles and cans of soft drink) for the training session. They were dressed in the standard OPAL uniform, a pink short-sleeved top with the OPAL logo embroidered onto the top left corner and slacks. Both women were in their mid- to late 20s, slim, and described as "glowing with health" by several attendees. Other participants in the room had a range of health problems (from decaying teeth to cancer), and many described themselves as "plump" (except for the man, who was thin).

Before the commencement of one of the early sessions, Scarlette had taped a poster (a handwritten sheet of cardboard) from last week to the wall. It listed the issues (identified the week before) that the group thought stopped them from eating healthily. After starting the day by talking about the importance of drinking water rather than soft drinks, Scarlette turned everyone's attention to the list and asked if anyone had anything to add to it. She then read out the issues one by one and drew in some comments from the participants. "So the first issue identified," says Scarlette is "lack of time." "What can we say about this?" One woman spoke about how having children makes time limited. Another said caring as a volunteer or "for other people in her life" made it harder for her to find the time to eat healthily.

The next item on the list was "lack of money." Some people commented that it was much cheaper to buy unhealthy food, like frozen pizzas, or buy take-out than it was to buy fresh vegetables. They commented on the affordability of a $10 family pizza at the local shops, or the ease at crossing the road to the service station for chocolate and chips. If participants didn't have a car, this was the easiest, and often only, option.

One woman said that organic food is around five to six times more expensive than non-organic food and you could never trust whether it is really organic anyway: "I don't know how to tell if something is truly organic, do you?" she asked the woman sitting next to her, who replied with a shrug of her shoulders while shaking her head. Rachel, then called out: "There are a lot of people with not much money in our community; people live on a lot less here."

"Then there is lack of knowledge," says Scarlette. "Does anyone have anything to say about this?" "You have to learn about what is really healthy first," said one participant. There was a list of things on the cardboard under this point, including "Limited skills to cook and prepare food," and "Social isolation." The very last point was "Not putting self first." The woman next to Tanya leaned over and said: "I can relate to that. I look after everyone else and then I'm happy with just a piece of toast." We thought it interesting that the lack of knowledge point was emphasized more than the first two, and wondered how much of the emphasis came from OPAL and how much came from community members themselves. Overall, the sessions stressed nutritional literacy and food hygiene—and ignored the relational aspects of food, eating, and care and how they intersect.

Caring is an important and overlooked role in food and eating, and it is women and mothers who disproportionally take on this role (Warin et al. 2008; Maher et al. 2010; Wright et al. 2015). Caring involves food work for children and families (planning meals, packing lunchboxes, cooking, shopping) and all manner of activities around the emotional investment of women in managing family eating. This gendered division of food work "rests on the shoulders of those who perform caring labor—namely women" (Carney 2015, p. 11), and is devalued as a form of social reproductive labor. We return to this theme of care and gendered relationships in the context of food in our next chapter.

At a graduation event held at the end of the training sessions Tanya talks to Meredith, a local healthcare worker. The conversation turns to recent changes in how community programs now run. "Ah well, Tanya there's not so much now. In the past there was heaps of stuff going on, really good programs, but now it's all dried up, it's been cut back and there isn't much of anything good left." "What do you mean?" Tanya asks. "Well," she says

> the whole approach is different now, and all the resources are so much tighter. We used to go into the community houses and get a whole bunch of people together, then we'd sit with them and listen and ask them what's important to them, what they want to see happen in their community, and that's how it'd go—the community would lead the programs and it was great. Now it's the total reverse. We get directed by SA Health. It's really top-down, like SA Health, the Health Promotion Branch, they want everything to be about obesity. They want us to tell the community that they are fat, that they're obese. To tell the parents they are fat and that their kids are fat too and that they need to lose weight. I'm serious, this is what it's like now. And so here we have OPAL and the other programs and that's the way it's become. SA Health tell us that we've got OPAL or we've got this or that. It's all top-down.

Tanya listens to Meredith intently, even if a little cautiously because of the two OPAL staff who were wandering around. Tanya whispers: "So, Meredith, where's the consultation? Is there any community consultation?" Meredith laughs incredulously: "Not a chance … there's none. There is no community consultation." Tanya asks: "How did it all become so top-down?" Meredith makes sure Scarlette is out of earshot:

> Well, look at OPAL. That's what we've come down to. These people come in here from outside the community, without a clue of what it's like to live in poverty, to have real social issues, low levels of education … and then they

stand up there and tell people to do this and to be that. I mean, get real! How bloody condescending is that? How patronizing, like they're idiots. What do you expect them to think? What do you expect them to say? How about 'fuck off!' So when Poppy was all shocked after the behavioral change evaluation when she found there wasn't any 'behavior change,' no impact, and then she's all surprised because there hadn't been *any* change from the OPAL program! I had to laugh. I mean, really, what the hell do you expect? When the Foodies trainers phone up people after these sessions, and ask them what they thought of the program, and they're just trying to get their kids out of bed or just struggling with life, you know, the issues … can't pay the bills … can't keep their house … like, how relevant is all of *this* to them, really? What do *you* think their priorities should be?" She paused. "I'm glad you're here Tanya. I think that there's a lot an anthropologist could do here.

* * *

In this chapter we have highlighted how assumptions about a knowledge deficit, the "right" way to eat, and romantic complexity all lead to a focus on individual behaviors. These types of interventions are cheap and comparatively easy to implement, and "rely on established idioms and ways of thinking" (Sanabria 2016, p. 135). Coupled with the "the moral millstone" (Coveney 2006) that is hung around the necks of those experiencing disadvantage, people are positioned as both ignorant and responsible at the same time. By spreading messages about healthy eating, and imparting nutritional knowledge and information they will learn how to eat "good, wholesome foods" and see through the hype of junk food advertising. OPAL thus presented healthy eating as a battle between two different types of knowledge—between expert "knowing" and lay "not-knowing." It was the "not-knowing" that needed to be corrected, and this was the premise of community education events in which bad eating habits could be transformed into good eating habits. In her comparison of EPODE in France and OPAL in Australia, Hartwick (2014) argues that OPAL was very attuned to "good" and "bad" foods, demonstrating that foods and eating were characterized within fairly conservative discourses that emanated from the efforts of governments and public health practitioners in the 1960s, telling people to avoid or reduce particular nutrients (Dixon 2016, p. 1115). It wasn't that all OPAL workers were ignorant of broader social determinants, but the overall template they were given meant they had to follow a script and didn't allow for wider types of engagement.

What was entirely overlooked was the diverse range of understandings about food and eating that preexisted in the community, not only local understandings but also other competing discourses that people turned to. Julie Guthman (2014) notes that hegemonic discourses are no longer the purview of dietitians and nutritionists. What is interesting are the distrust of scientific expert discourses and the dismantling of hierarchical knowledge. Now almost anyone can be an expert—celebrities (Gwyneth Paltrow), the media, food bloggers (including disgraced Australian wellness blogger Belle Gibson),[2] celebrity chefs (Jamie Oliver, Anthony Bourdain), and even friends and families (Guthman 2014).[3] OPAL often justified its rationale as "knowledge based on science," thereby excluding the wealth of lay knowledge that local community members had about food and eating or, indeed, many other avenues of public knowledge. These multiple registers of knowledge were not valued.

Health and the pursuit of healthism was not always a priority for people in the community, but stretching household food budgets and meals usually was. While OPAL wanted to get rid of minced meat from local supermarkets and the food bank and replace it with "healthier choices and leaner cuts," local people told us with great pride the many things you could do with mince. Ellie, who described herself as "dirt poor" when raising her two children, said:

> *There's a lot you can do with mince, believe me, loads of meals … meatballs, meatloaf, spaghetti Bolognese, shepherds pie, stewed mince. … I might get four meals out of 500 grams of mince—sometimes five … it's only about two dollars a meal. I always did all the cooking and I budgeted very well because we didn't have much money.*

OPAL, however, wanted to change the Spaghetti Bolognese and other meal packs sold at the food banks, many of which were deemed to be "not healthy" because they included cheap (rather than lean) cuts of meat, minimal vegetables, and flavor sachets (containing sugar and salt).

Ellie and other participants didn't lack knowledge about what to eat or how to cook and were proud of how they could make meals and finances stretch. Money, not health, was often the main priority in households and people made do within the constraints of limited budgets. In this context of tight budgets pleasure was highly valued, and the next chapter turns to the power and pleasures of sweetness.

Notes

1. An older brother of John Kellogg—Dr. Merritt Kellogg—designed the Sydney Sanitarium, which was opened in the suburbs of northern Sydney in 1903. Known today as the Sydney Adventist Hospital but referred to as the "The San," this large private hospital combines the missionary passion of spiritual healing and medical science.
2. Belle Gibson is a young Australian woman who in 2015 claimed to have cured her terminal brain cancer through adoption of a healthy diet. She personally profited through book contracts, an app (The Whole Food Pantry), and numerous charity appearances. The Federal Court of Australia found her guilty of misleading and deceptive conduct for falsely claiming she had cancer which was cured by alternative therapies and nutrition.
3. Evidence of this shift in trust to celebrities is documented by Jones et al. (2011, 2013), who found that in the UK more than 75% of the general population believed celebrity chefs promoted healthy eating and that their recipes were healthy (2011). Following up on this study, Jones et al. (2013) examined the nutritional content of 904 recipes from celebrity chef books and websites, finding that "[t]he majority of recipes analysed had unhealthy nutritional compositions [saturated fatty acids, sugar and salt] according to national healthy eating benchmark recommendations, and that therefore, celebrity chefs could potentially be a hidden contributory factor to current public health nutrition issues, through exacerbating Britain's already unbalanced dietary intake" (2013, p. 108).

References

Australian Bureau of Statistics. (2013). *Australian Health Survey: Updated results 2011–2012.* Cat no. 4364.0.55.003, Canberra.

Baum, F. (2011). From Norm to Eric: Avoiding lifestyle drift in Australian health policy. *Australian and New Zealand Journal of Public Health, 35*, 404–406.

Baum, F., & Fisher, M. (2014). Why behavioral health promotion endures despite its failure to reduce health inequities. *Sociology of Health and Illness, 36*(2), 213–225.

Bita, N. (2013, August 3). *The Advertiser.*

Bronfenbrenner, U. (1977). Toward an experimental ecology of human development. *American Psychologist, 32*, 513–531.

Carey, G., Malbon, E., Crammond, B., Pescud, M., & Baker, P. (2017). Can the sociology of social problems help us to understand and manage 'lifestyle drift'? *Health Promotion International, 32*(4), 755–761.

Carney, M. A. (2015). *Unending hunger.* Oakland: University of California Press.

Cohn, S. (2014). From health behaviors to health practices: An introduction. *Sociology of Health and Illness, 36*(2), 157–162.

Coveney, J. (1999). The science and spirituality of nutrition. *Critical Public Health, 9*(1), 23–37.

Coveney, J. (2006). *Food, morals and meaning: The pleasure and anxiety of eating* (2nd ed.). London: Routledge.

Coveney, J. (2008). The government of girth. *Health Sociology Review, 17*, 199–213.

Crawford, R. (1980). Healthism and the medicalization of everyday life. *International Journal of Health Services, 10*(3), 365–388.

Dehghan, M., Akhtar-Danesh, N., & Merchant, A. (2005). Childhood obesity, prevalence and prevention. *Nutrition Journal, 4*(1), 24.

Dixon, J. (2016). Critical nutrition studies within critical agrarian studies: A review and analysis. *The Journal of Peasant Studies, 43*(5), 1112–1120.

Evans, J., Davies, B., & Rich, E. (2008). The class and cultural functions of obesity discourse: Our latter day child saving movement. *International Studies in Sociology of Education, 18*(2), 117–132.

Farrell, L. C., Warin, M., Moore, V. M., & Street, J. M. (2016). Socio-economic divergence in public opinions about preventive obesity regulations: Is the purpose to 'make some things cheaper, more affordable' or to 'help them get over their own ignorance'? *Social Science and Medicine, 154*, 1–8.

Foucault, M. (1990). *The history of sexuality: Volume 1, an introduction.* Harmondsworth: Penguin.

Gard, M., & Wright, J. (2005). *The obesity epidemic: Science, morality and ideology.* London: Routledge.

Guthman, J. (2011). *Weighing in: Obesity, food justice and the limits of capitalism.* Berkeley: University of California Press.

Guthman, J. (2014). Introducing critical nutrition: A special issue on dietary advice and its discontents. *Gastronomica: The Journal of Critical Food Studies, 14*(3), 1–4.

Hartwick, C. (2014). *Transferring an innovation in food and lifestyle education: Development of a French childhood obesity prevention program in Australia. A cultural comparison of childhood obesity prevention in France and Australia.* Unpublished PhD thesis, Université Paris Descartes Ecole doctorale SHS (ED180) CERLIS/Education et Formation and Flinders University School of Public Health, Adelaide.

Hayes-Conroy, A., & Hayes-Conroy, J. (Eds.). (2013). *Doing nutrition differently: Critical approaches to diet and dietary intervention.* Surrey: Ashgate.

Hunter, D. J., Popay, J., Tannahill, C., & Whitehead, W. (2010). Getting to grips with health inequalities at last? *British Medical Journal, 340*, 323.

Ingold, T. (2013). Foreword. *Education in the North, 20*(Special Issue), 1. Retrieved from https://www.abdn.ac.uk/eitn/documents/Volume%20 20%20Special%20Issue/EITN%20Volume%2020%20foreword.pdf

Jones, M., Hennessey-Priest, K., & Costa, R. J. S. (2011). Do United Kingdom based celebrity chefs contribute to the current obesity epidemic and associated co-morbidities? *Annals of Nutrition and Metabolism, 58*, 387–388.

Jones, M., Freeth, E. C., Hennessy-Priest, K., & Costa, R. J. (2013). A systematic cross-sectional analysis of British based celebrity chefs' recipes: Is there cause for public health concern? *Food and Public Health, 3*(2), 100–110.

Kelly, M. P., & Russo, F. (2018). Causal narratives in public health: The difference between mechanisms of aetiology and mechanisms of prevention in non-communicable diseases. *Sociology of Health & Illness, 40*(1), 82–99.

Kowal, E. (2015). *Trapped in the gap: Doing good in Indigenous Australia*. New York: Berghahn Press.

Kritchevsky, D. (1988). Dietary fiber. *Annual Review of Nutrition, 8*, 301–328.

Kwa, C. (2002). Romantic and baroque conceptions of complex wholes in the sciences. In J. Law & A. Mol (Eds.), *Complexities: Social studies of knowledge practices* (pp. 23–52). Durham: Duke University Press.

Landecker, H. (2011). Food as exposure: Nutritional epigenetics and the new metabolism. *BioSocieties, 6*(2), 167–194.

Law, J. (2004). And if the global were small and noncoherent? Method, complexity, and the baroque. *Environment and Planning D: Society and Space, 22*(1), 13–26.

Lupton, D. (2014). 'How do you measure up?' Assumptions about "obesity" and health-related behaviors and beliefs in two Australian "obesity" prevention campaigns. *Fat Studies, 3*(1), 32–44.

Maher, J., Fraser, S., & Wright, J. (2010). Framing the mother: Childhood obesity, maternal responsibility and care. *Journal of Gender Studies, 19*(3), 233–247.

Mayes, C. (2016). *The biopolitics of lifestyle: Foucault, ethics and healthy choices*. New York: Routledge.

Mayes, C., & Thompson, D. (2015). What should we eat? Biopolitics, ethics, and nutritional scientism. *Bioethical Inquiry, 12*, 587–599.

Mol, A. (2012a). Layers or versions? Human bodies and the love of bitterness. In B. Turner (Ed.), *The Routledge handbook of the body* (pp. 119–129). Oxford/ New York: Routledge.

Mol, A. (2012b). Mind your plate! The ontonorms of Dutch dieting. *Social Studies of Science, 43*(3), 379–396.

Monaghan, L. F., Colls, R., & Evans, B. (2013). Obesity discourse and fat politics: Research, critique and interventions. *Critical Public Health, 23*(3), 249–262.

Obesity Australia. (2014). *Obesity: A national epidemic and its impact on Australia*. Sydney: Obesity Australia.

OPAL Collective. (2015). Practitioner insights on obesity prevention: The voice of South Australian OPAL workers. *Health Promotion International, 31*(2), 375–384.

Prentice, D. (2015). Targeting ignorance to change behavior. In M. Gross & L. McGoey (Eds.), *Routledge international handbook of ignorance studies* (pp. 266–273). London: Routledge.

Sanabria, E. (2016). Circulating ignorance: Complexity and agnogenesis in the obesity epidemic. *Cultural Anthropology, 31*(1), 131–158.

Schneidermann, N. (2018). Texting like a state: mHealth and the first thousand days in South Africa. Somatosphere. somatosphere.net/2018/01/texting-like-a-state.html

Scrinis, G. (2008). On the ideology of nutritionism. *Gastronomica, 8*(1), 39–48.

Scrinis, G. (2013). *Nutritionism: The science and politics of dietary advice.* New York: Columbia University Press.

Scrinis, G., & Parker, C. (2016). Front-of-pack food labeling and the politics of nutritional nudges. *Law & Policy, 38*(3), 234–249.

Shove, E., Pantzar, M., & Watson, M. (2012). *The dynamics of social practice: Everyday life and how it changes.* London: Sage.

Skrabanek, P. (1994). *The death of humane medicine and the rise of coercive healthism.* London: Social Affairs Unit.

Tuana, N. (2006). The speculum of ignorance: The women's health movement and epistemologies of ignorance. *Hypatia, 21*(3), 1–19.

Ulijaszek, S. (2015). With the benefit of foresight: Reframing the obesity problem as a complex system. *BioSocieties, 10*(2), 213–228.

Ulijaszek, S. J. (2017). *Models of obesity: From ecology to complexity in science and policy.* Cambridge: Cambridge University Press.

Ulijaszek, S., & McLennan, A. (2016). Framing obesity in UK policy from the Blair years, 1997–2015: The persistence of individualistic approaches despite overwhelming evidence of societal and economic factors, and the need for collective responsibility. *Obesity Reviews, 17*, 397–411.

Wang, G., & Dietz, W. (2002). Economic burden of obesity in youths aged 6 to 17 years: 1979–1999. *Pediatrics, 109*, e81.

Ward, P. J., Coveney, J., Verity, F., Carter, P., Tsourtos, G., & Wong, K. (2013). Food stress in Adelaide: The relationship between low income and the affordability of healthy food. *Journal of Environmental and Public Health*, 1–10. Available at http://www.hindawi.com/journals/jeph; https://doi.org/10.1155/2013/968078.

Warin, M. (2011). Foucault's progeny: Jamie Oliver and the art of governing obesity. *Social Theory and Health, 9*, 24–40.

Warin, M. (2018). Information is not knowledge: Cooking and eating as skilled practice in Australian obesity education. *The Australian Journal of Anthropology, 29*(1), 108–124.

Warin, M., Turner, K., Moore, V., & Davies, M. (2008). Bodies, mothers and identities: Rethinking obesity and the BMI. *Sociology of Health & Illness, 30*(1), 97–111.

Warin, M., Zivkovic, T., Moore, V., Ward, P. R. & Jones, M. (2015). Short horizons and obesity futures: Disjunctures between public health interventions and everyday temporalities. *Social Science & Medicine, 128*, 309–315.

Warin, M., Zivkovic, T., Moore, V., & Ward, P. (2017). Moral fiber: Breakfast as a symbol of 'a good start' in an Australian obesity intervention. *Medical Anthropology, 36*(3), 217–230.

White, E. (1905/2015). *The Ministry of healing*. Ellen G. White Estate, Inc. Available at https://egwwritings.org/media/pdf/en_MH.pdf

Wilson, B. C. (2014). *Dr. John Harvey Kellogg and the religion of biologic living*. Bloomington: Indiana University Press.

Wright, J., Maher, J., & Tanner, C. (2015). Social class, anxieties and mothers' foodwork. *Sociology of Health & Illness, 37*(3), 422–436.

Yates-Doerr, E. (2012). The opacity of reduction: Nutritional black-boxing and the meanings of nourishment. *Food, Culture and Society, 15*(2), 293–313.

Yates-Doerr, E. (2015). *The weight of obesity: Hunger and global health in postwar Guatemala*. Oakland: University of California Press.

Zivkovic, T., Warin, M., Davies, M., & Moore, V. (2010). In the name of the child: The gendered politics of childhood obesity. *Journal of Sociology, 46*, 375–392.

Zivkovic, T., Warin, M., Moore, V., Ward, P., & Jones, M. (2015). The sweetness of care: Biographies, bodies and place. In E. Abbotts, A. Lavis, & L. Attala (Eds.), *Careful eating: Bodies, food and care* (pp. 109–112). Farnham: Ashgate.

CHAPTER 5

Hide the Sugar!

You know you can buy a Maccas[1] *burger for two dollars, do you know what I'm saying? Like why wouldn't you? It's done, it's ready, it's delicious. So full of sugar and fat, it's really unhealthy, but it's two dollars.* (Candy)

In March 2016 Lucy Cormack, a crime reporter for the *Sydney Morning Herald*, wrote this headline: "Australia's sugar intake [is] described by experts as alarming."[2] Taking her data from a recently published academic paper on the dietary intake of added sugars in the Australian population (Lei et al. 2016), she reported that more than half of all Australians consume beyond the maximum recommended daily intake of added sugars. The worst offenders in this sugary overconsumption were said to be sugar-sweetened drinks (no brands named), followed by sweet spreads and cakes, biscuits, and pastries (Lei et al. 2016, p. 875). These beverages and items are often presented as "empty calories"—energy-dense and/or nutrient-poor discretionary foods. The study and media coverage concluded that young people aged 14–18 have the highest added sugar intake, thus making a case for targeting children and teenagers with messages about reducing their consumption of highly sweetened drinks. This published study was cited as an important addition to the field of knowledge, as there had been no update on Australia's sugar consumption for over 20 years, since the 1995 National Nutrition Survey.

We have to wonder why a crime reporter is writing about sugar, and you could argue that there are a number of clues in relation to the negative

M. Warin, T. Zivkovic, *Fatness, Obesity, and Disadvantage in the Australian Suburbs*,
https://doi.org/10.1007/978-3-030-01009-6_5

discourses and current demonization of sugar. Sugar is very much in the limelight as a key risk factor for diet-related diseases, like obesity and diabetes, and is touted in clinical, public health, and the popular press as "driving all of the chronic metabolic diseases that we know about today" (Lustig 2013a). It is represented as a "culprit" (Lim 2013), a "sweet poison" (Gillespie 2008), a "white powder" that is compared to morphine or heroin (Dufty 1975; c.f. Fischler 1987), a "dietary villain that's making us fat and sick" (Lustig 2013b; Kinshella 2017), and "toxic" (ABC *Catalyst*).[3] In a comparative ethnographic piece on sugar in Japan, Holtzman (2016) suggests that sugar is portrayed as "little different from an illicit drug … once you're hooked, you're hooked: and when you're hooked, you'll most likely put on weight, and probably a lot of it" (Holtzman 2016, p. 48).

Sugar hasn't always been in the limelight though. Professor of sociology, Marion Nestle, has led a sustained critique of the political machinations of the food industry and powerful corporate sectors to influence consumer behavior, academic research, and government legislation.[4] She argues that sugar, along with saturated fats, was clearly identified as a mortality risk factor in 1967. But up until very recently, "scientists and dietary guidelines focused on reducing saturated fat as the primary strategy for CHD [chronic heart disease] prevention" (Nestle 2016, p. 1686). The demonization of fat and the proliferation of low-fat consumables (e.g. low-fat yogurts, low-fat milk, low-fat cheeses, low-fat biscuits) led to sugar being added to make low-fat foods more palatable and, indeed, as a healthy alternative, driving higher consumption. Now that the incidence of obesity and diabetes has risen in the last four decades, health authorities are questioning if we were given the right advice. Sugar is now the "new fat" or the "new tobacco" (Atwell 2013), and people are encouraged to be wary of the stealth in which sugar operates. Sugar hides in foods, it dissolves in drinks, and is invisible to consumers. Participants in our study were told by Obesity Prevention and Lifestyle (OPAL) workers that sugar is so good at hiding that "sometimes you cannot even taste it." As the national UK obesity campaign Change4Life states, people now need to be "sugar smart."

This present focus on sugar as a major culprit in the obesity epidemic is currently at play on the international stage. The World Health Organization (WHO) has urged all countries to place a tax on sugary drinks in order to curb the "soaring obesity rates, especially in children." All eyes are on those countries (at the time of writing 26) that have introduced sugar or soda taxes. Mexico was one of the first, in 2014, adding a one peso per liter excise tax on drinks with added sugar. A follow-up study in 2016 (Colchero et al. 2017) showed an average reduction of 7.6% in the purchase of taxed sugary drinks during 2014 and 2015, with households with the fewest resources having an average reduction of 11.7% (WHO 2017). Other countries have followed suit (e.g. Ireland, South Africa, France, and Norway) and in April 2018 the UK Government introduced a sugar tax, enforcing soft drink manufacturers to pay a tax on sugary drinks.

Some sections of Australian society (including academics) are highly aware of this international wave to curb sugar consumption and have been lobbying the Australian Government to introduce a sugar tax. However, the government (and the heavily subsidized sugarcane industry in Queensland) continues to protest against a "moralistic tax on sugar," returning to arguments of personal responsibility. The former Deputy Prime Minister of Australia Barnaby Joyce in denying that a sugar tax would have any impact on obesity, suggested that Australians should "take responsibility on yourself … put on a pair of sandshoes and walk around the block … get yourself a robust chair and a heavy table and half-way through the meal put both hands on the table and just push back—that will help you lose weight" (Joyce 2017). This neoliberal approach to obesity, in which shame and guilt is directly linked to failures in personal responsibility, is something we come back to later on.

In this chapter we investigate the multiple meanings of sugar as they circulated in our field sites, through OPAL messages and in people's lives. We begin by looking at the ways in which sugar was presented to the community by the OPAL program, as a substance that caused harm and weight gain. Participants knew that sugar in clinical terms was deemed to be unhealthy, but this understanding existed alongside a host of meanings that were often more important in people's everyday lives. Sugar may be empty calories, but it is not an empty category.

Rather than focus on sugar as a thing, as a bad substance to drink or eat, we found that participants used sugar and sweetness to nourish social relationships. Following Mol's idea of care as a process of "tinkering" (2010; Mol et al. 2010a), which involves "crafting more bearable ways of living with, or in, reality" (Mol 2008, p. 53), we show how care is configured in the context of food, eating, and disadvantage. Sweetness, we argue, emerges as a strategy of caring (for oneself and for others) practiced by low-income families to negotiate social hierarchies and relations, and sweeten circumstances that have gone sour (Zivkovic et al. 2015). Families thereby reclaimed the meanings of sugar beyond a nutritional discourse of "dietary sugar," and "sweetness" permeated everyday language as people were described as "sweetie" or "honey," things were "sweet," and circumstances became palatable. As such, we view sweetness *as* a practice of care.

Moreover, being told that they were eating too much sugar, or having to cut back on sugar, left some community members affronted. This was not simply a response to what was perceived as a "top-down" obesity intervention, but rather resistance to the lack of choice that such moral overtures presented. Exercising choice in food consumption was key to people's sense of agency, and the food bank's philosophy upheld choice as more important than healthy options, which were seen to reduce people's choices and avenues to enjoy small pleasures. Sweetening is thus a useful conceptual category for thinking through the discordance between public health understandings of sugar and how ethnography reveals local contingencies of care and resistance through sweetness.

Sugar as "Bad"

Sugar has always been on the "only sometimes and in small amounts" list of the Australian Dietary Guidelines. In 2013, the guidelines advised Australians to limit their intake of foods and drinks containing "added sugars," as they are associated with weight gain and tooth decay (c.f. ABS 2016). The OPAL program similarly took sugar to task, noting that in Australia the highest per capita intake of soft drink consumption for children was in South Australia, and the greatest in "those children from families of lowest SES" (OPAL Fact Sheet). OPAL emphasized sugar consumption in three of their six social marketing campaigns (Water. The original cool drink; Make it a Fresh Snack; and A Healthy Brekky is easy as Peel, Pour, Pop). People in the community also acknowledged that sugar was implicated in ill-health, with one local worker from Reshaping Playford stating:

> *This community is disadvantaged. There is a long history of inadequate nutrition. It is not uncommon to see parents feeding their toddlers McDonalds® and the babies drinking Coke® from a bottle. There has been a lot of trouble with tooth decay among really, young kids.*

A preliminary survey conducted by OPAL in the area confirmed that soft drinks consumption was high. The penchant for sugary drinks and foods was seen as a behavior that needed to be changed in the community.

As well as installing two water fountains (one in a local community hub and another in a public park) and reducing the price of water below that of soft drinks in a local gym, OPAL staff began to work with the food banks and assess items for their sugar (and nutritional) content.

As one of the many identified stakeholder organizations in the community, the two food banks were key sites where OPAL operated. When OPAL staff started working in the food banks, the food selection began to change to healthier options and items high in sugar (such as cordial) occupied increasingly contested spaces. At the time of the "healthy breakfast" theme, an OPAL staff member suggested that OPAL-approved cereals be marked out in the shop by "shelf wobblers" (OPAL-endorsed labels) while unhealthy sugary cereals, in an attempt to reduce their consumption by poor families, should be priced higher. Volunteers told us that biscuits and sugary drinks were also "not OPAL-approved," and there was a push from OPAL to change ingredients of the prepackaged kids school and kindergarten packs that were made and sold in the food banks to have "water instead of juice, and no sweet biscuits, muesli bars, chocolate or chips." "We've got to be a bit educational" says Katie, the local volunteer. "We're not allowed to sell things like Coke®." We asked if more customers would come and if they would buy more food from the food bank if they sold Coke®: "I'm sure they would; certainly more people would buy from us."

Guess the Sugar

The first OPAL social marketing theme that was endorsed by the Scientific Advisory Committee began in 2010 and was entitled *Water—the original cool drink*. The "behavior target" around the marketing of this theme was to encourage children to choose water instead of sweet drinks (e.g. soft drinks, fruit drinks, cordial, flavored mineral waters, sports drinks, energy drinks, and fruit juice). All leaflets and brochures listed reasons for switching to water, always health-related warnings (tooth decay or excess weight gain), with some brochures also emphasizing the money that could be saved by drinking tap water rather than purchasing heavily marketed commercial products.

Accompanying the shift to healthy and cheap drinks was a ubiquitous education theme: Guess the Sugar. In brochures this was a pictorial representation showing how many teaspoons of sugar were in a drink. Guess the Sugar was set up at many OPAL events—at Community Foodies training days, at local schools, in public places (outside the local library),

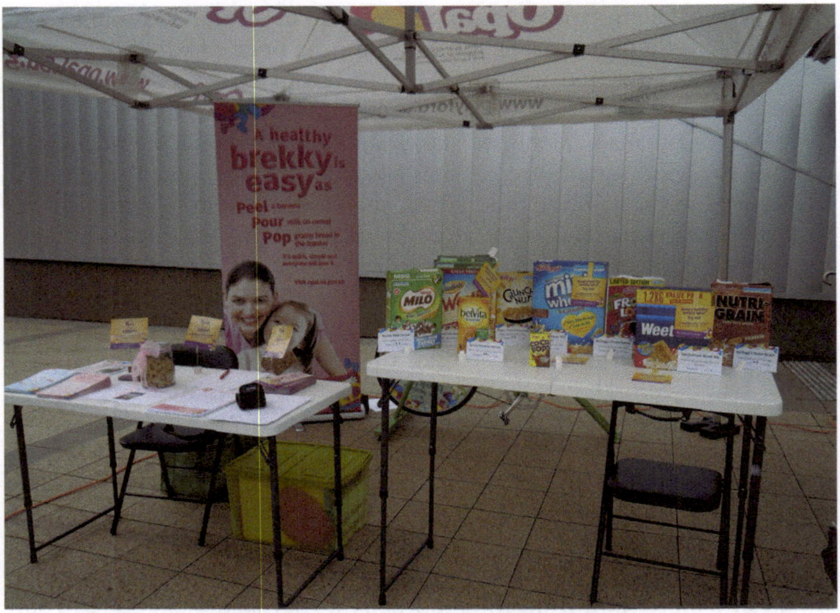

Fig. 5.1 "Guess the Sugar" display at the local shopping center. (Photo from Authors)

and in community centers. In this game a range of popular drinks (including Coke®, iced coffee, Monster® [an "energy" drink], and Mount Franklin® water), and sometimes breakfast cereals, were lined up and the demonstrator asked the audience to guess how much sugar there was in each one, or to rank the sugar content (Fig. 5.1).

At one Community Foodies session with the local Burundian (East African) community, the instructor, Faith, showed pictures of drinks to the group. There was a page containing 600 ml bottles of Coke®, Diet Coke®, Sprite®, and Fanta®. She asked the group to guess which contained the most sugar before telling them that Fanta did. She turned the page over to reveal the number of teaspoons each contained, and the ten Burundian men and women looked shocked at the amount of sugar there was in every drink except Diet Coke®. "How is there no sugar in Diet Coke® when it tastes so sweet?" asked Nella, the Burundian interpreter. Faith tells her that it contains an artificial sweetener. She goes on:

"But this fake sugar is not good for you either. The latest research shows that this artificial sugar makes you hungry. It tricks your body and the body thinks that there is sugar coming and so it gets really hungry and causes people to eat more, so it is best to avoid the sweeteners. They are a sometimes drink but it's best if you avoid them."

The next picture showed Red Bull® and Mother®. Faith stated that Red Bull® contains 6 teaspoons of sugar and Mother contains 11. "These drinks are high in sugar and they are also bad for your heart." The next page showed some milk drinks. "The 600 ml iced coffee has 11.5 teaspoons of sugar and two teaspoons of fat. The 600 ml Classic Chocolate Milk® has 11 teaspoons of sugar and three teaspoons of fat. The Feel Good® iced coffee has three teaspoons of sugar and one teaspoon of fat." Again, the faces of the women in the group dropped. "Are you surprised by this?" asked the other instructor. It was clear by their faces that they were not happy with the news. "We're not telling you to stop but we are just showing you how much fat and sugar they contain. So, if you are drinking these drinks and you are putting on a few extra kilos you can probably see why that could happen." Nella says "I am addicted to Fanta® and Coke®. I just don't think I could give them up. I can't stop." "You don't have to stop but you could try to reduce. Baby steps," says Amy. "OK, I'll slowly reduce, slowly," says Nella, with a sigh.

This surprise or shock value is key to the pedagogical element of the exercise. In OPAL and other community health education spaces sugar is discursively constructed as a significant problem. It is *only* represented as negative, as a "bad" and malevolent entity that hides in foods and drinks unbeknownst to the consumer. In "outing" how many teaspoons of sugar are in sugary drinks, it is assumed that people will then "know better" and change their behaviors. This strategy is helped by marketing sugar as a dangerous substance that can, as Amy explains to the group, "cause chronic disease later in life, including high blood pressure, diabetes, heart disease, and some types of cancer." At the end of the session described earlier, and when everyone had left the room, the instructors turned to each other: "Did you see their faces when I told them how much sugar were in the take-away foods and the soft drinks? … I've never seen such sad faces before when I've given that information. I really feel sorry for them. At the end they said 'Thank you' and that 'It's good to know these things' but at the time they looked really horrified, didn't they?"

This device of instilling fear is often used in public health campaigns (early HIV campaigns, smoking, and diabetes). The logic is that in showing people the risks, through a "semiotics of fear," certain behaviors will be deterred. Brookes and Harvey argue that

> *despite the documented benefits of using more positive appeals to promote health, employing, for example, supportive messages that underscore hope, reward, and positive consequences* (Hastings et al. 2004; Rothman et al. 2006), *arguably the most common (and certainly the most controversial) strategy used in recent times is that of scare tactics—discourses designed to create fear and anxiety in people* (Hastings et al. 2004; Hill et al. 1998). (Brookes and Harvey 2015, p. 61)

Fear is used as a common tactic in mass media public health campaigns as it is seen to be attention-grabbing and to shock people into behavior change (Borland and Balmford 2003). The 1987 AIDS media campaign in Australia is a classic case in point. Personifying AIDS as "the grim reaper," the deathly figure rolled a heavy, black ball down a bowling alley and knocked down innocent members of a family standing as pins. This mass media campaign was designed with the clear intent of (mis)representing AIDS as a contagious (rather than sexually transmitted) disease and frightening the Australian public (Lupton 2013). Similarly, graphic images on Australian cigarette packets featuring mouth cancer, gangrenous toes, and lungs clogged with black tar and cancer were designed to provoke emotional responses of disgust and fear, hoping to evoke visceral responses to scare people into behavioral change.

Brookes and Harvey suggest that researchers in public health have found that such fear-arousing health messages are "more likely to be effective when the message recipients have a high degree of self-efficacy" (2015, p. 61). People who have the resources and are "better placed, socially and psychologically, to respond to persuasive messages" (ibid.) are more likely to act on public health messages and benefit from their capacity to make changes. People who are less resourced, and less socially and psychologically able, often find that such messages make them feel worse, and reinforce a sense of failure. This was Fred's experience of the OPAL messaging. As a 25-year-old unemployed man he says that "[OPAL] made me feel like I'm not doing enough … [as if I am] lazy … it's a demotivating feeling." Or, as we go on to explain in this chapter, the tactics could engender resentment and resistance to all messages about healthy eating. While the instructors talked to the Burundian women about the dangers of diabetes and cardiovascular disease in light of the weight they had put on since migrating to Australia five or six years ago, none of this was contextualized in the cultural nuances of African bodies and eating, or the complexities of nutritional transition (Popkin 2001).

Circulations of Sweetness

Sugar, as anthropologist Mintz's classic history of sugar beautifully illustrates, is more than a metabolic source of energy. Mintz traces the shifting fortunes of sugar—how the European and American colonies transformed it from a little-known substance in medieval times to a luxury item available to the wealthy, and then to a necessity that by the nineteenth century formed a staple food for the British working classes (Holtzman 2016, p. 48; Mintz 1986). Throughout these changing eras, sugar has been regarded variously as a precious commodity, an everyday necessity, a preservative, a medicine, confectionary decoration, a spice or condiment, and a sweetener. Sugar has different inflections, depending on historical and cultural contexts, and has held a key place in mass consumption and in the capitalist system of labor exploitation and food production. Within this history, the "vulgarization" of sugar, or what Fischler calls "saccharophobia" (1987, p. 13), is a comparatively modern phenomenon.

Of note is the title of Mintz's book *Sweetness and Power* rather than *Sugar and Power*. Sugar is only one form of sweetness and Mintz was interested in why the desire for sweetness was historically so widespread and intense. Sweetness encompasses political economy, emotion, and affect, and the taste of sweetness has a distinctive history that influenced not only diets in the West, but was intimately entangled with notions of race, gender, and class, as well as the sense of self—especially in relation to family, community, and labor. Building on this history of sweetness, anthropologists using sensory approaches (Seremetakis 1994; Stoller 1989) have similarly shown how sweetness is entangled in social relations. For example, Cowan (1991) and Warin and Dennis (2005) have demonstrated how sweetness and the senses are deeply entwined, in that the apparently natural or taken-for-granted sensory practices of encountering sugar (e.g. eating it, tasting it, smelling it, seeing it) are invested with meaning, emotion, memory, and value. Fragrant hot black tea sucked through lumps of hard Persian sugar connect otherwise distant sites of Iranian homes in social custom, past and present (Warin and Dennis 2005). The ingestion of locally produced fruit-flavored liqueur in Greece, served in "a richly adorned thin-stemmed glass [of] silver or crystal," enables Sohoian "girls and women [to] literally produce themselves as properly feminine persons" (Cowan 1991, pp. 65–66).

In our field site sugar and sweetness had multiple registers. On the first day that Tanya began volunteering work at one of the food banks, the manager, gave her instructions to familiarize herself with the stock. "Now Tanya, you just have a look around and acquaint yourself with where some of the things are. You can start to stock up some of the shelves, like some of the bags of sugar … that is always a big seller. We always have to restock the sugar."

This unassuming, white, cheap product was a dominant item in the food banks and no less in people's lives. While instant coffee, tomato sauce, milk, and sausages were obvious staples, the food bank shelves were also filled with sugary cereals (Coco Pops®, Nutri-Grain®), cordial, biscuits, jams, and chocolate spreads. Sweet foods and drinks not only tasted good but were purchased and eaten as a treat, as a reward for good behavior, or to soften the hard knocks of lives. One day at the food bank, a mother yelled out to her late-teen daughters in delight at seeing single serves of jam: "I love these! We get these in jail!" After spending her $40 voucher from the Salvos [Salvation Army], she opens the packet of chocolate Oreo biscuits just purchased, and hands some to her toddler in a stroller: "Here you are lovely; you have been so good for us while we've been shopping. You've been such a good girl in there." As is well documented, sweet foods are often used to reward children for "being good" (McLennan et al. 2014).

Sweetening was a way to comfort and connect through momentary pleasures, and people would sometimes come into the food bank openly seeking a "pick-me-up." One morning a young man wearing a tattered black coat came into the shop, shaking as he spoke: "I just want something to cheer me and my mum up. I've got $3." From behind the counter Katie asked him: "How about some biscuits? Biscuits cheer everyone up don't they?" "Oh yes, I think you're right there. They do tend to cheer mum up … and me too." The young man then spent all his money on biscuits: Rocky Road biscuits for $1, Honeycomb Tim Tams® for 75 cents, and white chocolate Tim Tams® for 50 cents.

As well as "cheering up" lives, the sweet taste of sugar often takes precedence over the knowledge that too much sugar is "bad for diabetes." Jan commented on the "ballooning weight" of June, one of the regular volunteers at the food bank. "She's getting bigger and bigger. She has put on a lot of weight since she started here. I know I'm fat but June, well, she is as wide as she is tall. She's four by four." June was a diabetic and staff constantly worried about her health. They'd call out to each other across the shop: "Where's June? Anyone seen June?" After June was found coming back from the toilet, Jan told us: "June is diabetic but she's got no idea how to manage her diabetes and she has lots of hypos. No matter how many times she's been told, she's still eating all the wrong foods. So we've got to keep an eye on her, look after her because she can just go into a hypo at any moment." A month later, when offered chocolates around Easter time, June reminded everyone how she shouldn't be eating chocolate: "I can't have one—well, I shouldn't. But I do sometimes eat chocolate. I can't help it. I really like it."

Traveling around the field sites on public transport, Tanya would often hear conversations about the dangers of sugar, sometimes between strangers just making conversation with each other between their bus or train stops. Sitting on the bus one day, Tanya could not help but overhear a woman's conversation with an elderly man and woman who were sitting on different seats and did not appear to know each other. She wrote in her field notes:

> *The woman who is talking seems to be in her fifties, she is overweight, perhaps clinically obese, and she has to talk loudly at times for the elderly couple who are hard of hearing. "Oh I don't know what to do with my daughter. She is such a worry. You see she is diabetic and she takes no care of herself. She'll just eat a box of chocolates for dinner or lollies.[5] She's always eating bloody lollies. It's gonna do her in if she keeps up like this. She's got depression too. When she comes over to my place to stay she is all like she doesn't want to do anything. Just sit and mope about watching tele and eating lollies … I don't know what to do with her. I tell her 'If you give up girl, that'll be it. Don't you give up girl. Buck up!'" The woman continues after she rings the bell and stands up to get off the bus … "'You see this here stick', I tell her, 'Well you know what I'm gonna have to do if you don't give up'."*
>
> *A young toddler (about 18 months old) sits in a pram eating from a brown paper McDonald's bag while his mum drinks a large soft drink from McDonald's. Empty soft drink bottles rattle around the floor of the bus.*

These examples demonstrate not only the ubiquity of sugar but the multiple enactments sweetness has in this community. It is a commodity—a "big seller" in the food banks—a reward for children, a comfort, and a source of pleasure: at the same time it is a danger to health and a product that ends up as rubbish on a bus.

In our interviews with people, and our observations from volunteering in the food banks, we were struck by how much people talked about sweetness. Lyn, an overweight mother of five children who survives on government benefits, told us her body "craves sweet things." She said "I really try to be healthy and to not eat crap but you know I've got a sweet tooth and sometimes when things really get under my skin, I'll think to myself, 'Go on then, have some chocolate'." As recent research on care and food has elucidated, sugar is "not only the *substance*, food that has value" (e.g. nutritional value) but "the *practice*, eating, is at least as important" (Mol 2010, p. 217, [original emphasis]). Here the immediate pleasures of food prompt Lyn to take time out to care for herself.

When we discussed our research findings on the pleasures of sweetness, the OPAL manager said to us: "But everyone likes sweet things, everyone likes chocolate." Our research, however, demonstrated that sweetness needed to be understood within a socioeconomic context and the social gradient of obesity (Warin et al. 2015; Zivkovic et al. 2015). We found, as did Bissell et al. (2016) in their research with disadvantaged families in South Yorkshire, that eating was for pleasure and survival, not just for health (Warin et al. 2015, p. 314) and that food pleasures were woven into acts of caring, providing "a sense of well-being that spreads out for a moment, not a projection toward a future" (Berlant 2011, p. 117). Food pleasure is affordable, accessible, immediate, and reliable in a way that other pleasures are not (Bissell et al. 2016; Pampel 2012). In short, the immediate pleasures of food, and particularly of sweetness, were germane to our participants' everyday practices and an understandable response to their stressful environments.

Caring for Oneself

Caring for oneself by eating sweet foods is associated in our participants' narratives with cravings, desires, and their fulfillment, but also with unwanted weight gain and health problems. Bissell et al. (2016) refer to this struggle over the pleasures of foods and the struggle for control over eating as "discordant pleasures" (2016, p. 16). These contrasting and at times competing experiences of sugar consumption and its effects are apparent in the disclosure of an 18-year-old participant, Sienna. Describing herself as "skinny, but a little pudgy," Sienna says parts of her body are "very flabby" and she conceals her arms and stomach, admitting that she never wears tee shirts although she is fond of sporting tight stockings or long socks under short skirts.

Sienna has a history of what she terms "severe depression and anxiety" and reports being a "fussy eater" since the age of four. She is disgusted by the taste of vegetables, she dislikes most meats, salads make her shudder, she despises the smell of mushrooms, can't eat nuts, won't touch seafood, rarely eats bread, avoids spicy food, hates the taste of milk, abhors rice, and doesn't eat eggs. In our first interview, Sienna revealed that her self-described "fussiness" emerged after her parents' separation when she was around two and that it intensified in the course of a custody battle, after which her father moved interstate for a decade, an event which she says she is "still reeling from." She says: "I had no control over my life except for what I could eat because of all the custody drama, you know. I didn't feel in control. So, I would pick what I ate. And it's just kind of stuck with me." It is not only the avoidance of some foods that forms part of Sienna's coping strategy, learned from an early age, for dealing with the vicissitudes of her life. Conversely, the taste of certain other foods is equally important and associated with pleasure and social cohesion. When asked what she does to get by when stressful things happen to her, Sienna says she eats "comfort foods."

While pleasure is constrained in Sienna's household by physical illness and psychological distress, sweetness is easily gained through the consumption of "junk food like chocolate, chips, anything your heart desires and craves at that moment, you know, soft drinks ... because if you're stressed out, you kind of need something. [You say] I deserve this. This is going to help me. Usually, for me, it's comfort food." While sweetening social life through sugary foods is a practice Sienna uses to comfort and care for herself, she also positions sugar as dangerous:

> *Hey, I got to stop this "cause if I keep doing this I'm gonna get really fat, and that's really bad ... because you know, the larger you are, the more chance that, you know, the higher chance of you developing diabetes or, you know, being overweight means there's a few years cut off your life, you know?"*

Yet Sienna's knowledge about the harmful effects of sugar and fat does not instigate a change in her eating practices. Observing a higher prevalence of obesity in her neighborhood, Sienna commented: "Everything is just really crap around here it's like you just want to comfort eat 'cause everything sucks, so ... yeah."

Consuming sugar for Sienna can be an active agent in achieving moments of pleasure and comfort, candy-coating bitter circumstances, and sweetness can be embodied and experienced as self-care in the consumption of sweet foods. Sweet foods become a performance of care of the self, and for Sienna, and many other participants, eating was "a form of ballast against wearing out" (Berlant 2011, p. 116).

Relishing comfort foods is also an act of resistance against the public health imperative of healthy eating. Chocolates are sometimes squirreled away, hidden in Sienna's bedroom, and eaten in secret. Enacted at night, either in the privacy of her bedroom or with her mother in the living room, "comfort eating" is a way to sweeten the stressors of day-to-day social life: the threat of violent neighbors, financial insecurity, and the routine of acting out social pleasantries in her poorly paid, part-time, and precarious customer service job at a local hardware store. To Sienna, people who "come through my register and steal things" or who are "just so rude" and neighbors who can become violent and who threaten "to bash me with a metal pole" are part and parcel of living in the area. "Everyone up here is so rude. And like, in the city they're kind of snobby, but at least they're nice if you talk to them. Here it's like, 'I hate you because you looked at me funny!'"

Care for Others: Social Relations

While sweetness is often used and marketed toward care for the self, it is also a critical ingredient in our care for others. Rewarding children with lollipops and ice cream, demonstrating appreciation or adoration with a box of chocolates, and celebrating the progression of others' years with a birthday cake are culturally normative exchanges that sweeten social relations. This sweetening of social life is played out in the relationship between Sienna and her mother, with whom she lives.

Having ironically chosen the pseudonym Candy, Sienna's mother describes purchasing the foods that lighten her daughter's moments of anxiety and depression. Candy's identity is intricately related to her position as a mother. Having moved out of her natal home at the age of 13, Candy enjoys being the caretaker and provider for her 18-year-old daughter and also nurtures other young boarders who share her home. Candy buys the foods she knows Sienna will eat and drink: usually sweet-tasting soft drinks, processed pasta sachets, and biscuits. Much of Sienna's socializing occurs at night at home with her mother and house boarder, sitting in front of the television, where they chat, and enjoy the pleasures of sharing around sweet foods. In this household snacking is often restrained during the day but, as Sienna explains,

> *[a]fter dinner it's like fair game. Everyone is just like SNACK! If we're, you know, if we're sitting in the lounge and we're like, "I feel like a snack," then we get up. And then like an hour later someone else would be like, "I feel like a snack," and then someone will bring back other things.*

In Candy and Sienna's lounge room the experience of sweetness operates to strengthen social relations through the sharing of taste, and also by making time and space for its consumption (McLennan et al. 2014). The consumption of sweet foods, like cigarettes before them, demarcates liminal zones where everyday concerns are temporarily suspended (in tea breaks, "smokos,"[6] and snack times) and where commodities are fetishized and enjoyed.

Graham (1994), in her influential study on gender and class as dimensions of smoking behavior in Britain, found that cigarette smoking was associated with women from lower socioeconomic classes who have caring responsibilities combined with limited financial resources. In her study, smoking punctuated the passing of time. It was a way of marking time and making time in an otherwise chaotic or tedious day. Making time in the day for oneself is promoted in the long-running Nestlé® slogan that consumers should "Have a break … have a Kit Kat®," enacting self-care through momentary pleasures. In a similar light, the Australian confectionary brand Allen's reminds us that pleasure and joy, despite difficult circumstances, can be experienced in the present; hence the marketing slogan: "It's moments like these you need Minties®."[7]

Like smoko breaks, snack time is processual, reproducing social relations night-by-night. This intimate and relational practice of snacking in front of the television can offer an escape from the stressors of life, where the commensality of being with others, either in the flesh or virtually on screen, is sweetened through sharing those foods and drinks that are promoted as being associated with "enjoyment and immediate gratification" (Harris et al. 2009). Sugary products may pose "risks" to health but they are advertised and promoted as a reward, a "happy, sometimes secretive or 'naughty' indulgence" (McLennan et al. 2014). Candy buys large packets containing "fun-sized chocolates" or single servings of sweet biscuits, such as Tiny Teddies®. Acknowledging that "[i]t's more expensive that way" she is paying heed to health advice, purchasing sugary foods "in small amounts," and in line with her daughter's desire to lose weight. "You know," Candy says, "[i]t's a moment on the lips, a lifetime on the hips." Competing paradigms of care collide as health discourses of "careful eating" and relational practices of sweetening shape and constrain food portions and preferences. However, restraint is difficult to exercise at night when "subversive" eating (Albon 2005) takes hold. As Sienna conveys guiltily, "[i]t's a bad system, I must admit. But that's what we do." Contested enactments of care are played out in Candy's relationship with her obese stepdad. While her own mother worries about his weight and its impact on his health, Candy sneaks him lollipops asserting that "[y]ou can't deny the man everything."

Participants' practices of care contrasted sharply with the care of self that was expected to be an outcome of OPAL's messages around reducing sugar intake (Warin et al. 2015). Anthropologists and care theorists have for some time highlighted the political malleability of "care": how care can be used to support different political agendas (Tronto 1993) that inform cultural imaginings of food and eating (cf. Mol 2010). Care, as it is employed in healthcare or healthy lifestyle programs, is embedded in culturally entrenched understandings of what is morally "right" and what is "good," both for bodies and for society (Barnes 2012; Held 2006). Eating "good" food and performing the "right" activities are valued by health interventions such as OPAL as ways to educate and support families to care for themselves and for others (by eating and sharing these "right" foods). As such, good intentions are implicit in these understandings of care (Mol et al. 2010b, p. 12) and are taken for granted in obesity prevention strategies. As this chapter demonstrates, however, this form of caring, which aims to stop people from eating and drinking substances that are cheap, plentiful, and tasty, misses its mark because asking people to refrain from one of the few things that make them feel good seems implicitly uncaring.

"Hide the Chocolate!"

OPAL workers were aware that asking people to take control and responsibility for their eating choices might make them appear to be "food Nazis" or the "food police." Certainly those working and volunteering in the food banks did feel under surveillance and there were power tussles over who knew the community and what "was best for people who used the food banks." There were extra layers of bureaucracy placed on the food bank managers ("efficiency" drives) and reporting back to the local council, who funded the service. One Thursday morning, coming into the food bank, Tanya immediately saw the Dove® dark chocolate sitting behind the counter and marked for sale at $1. "The food bank is selling chocolate?" Tanya asks Vivienne. "Yes, those are mine. They have sold out in the shop now. It went quick. Everyone was happy to see chocolate in here. It's the first time they've sold it, at least the first time since I've worked here. We are selling chocolate wafer biscuits too for a good price, 50 cents a packet." Tanya mentions the chocolate to Katie when she sees her: "Oh, please don't say anything to anyone. Don't tell my boss. That's what I've been saying to all the customers too when they come in here all excited about us having chocolate saying 'Wow, you've got chocolate now.' I say to them, 'Don't tell my boss!'"

The food bank workers felt they had to keep the chocolate a secret, as they knew they would face increased scrutiny from OPAL and the local council. Once the other food bank heard on the grapevine that chocolates were for sale, they were emboldened to do the same. Favorite Australian chocolate biscuits, Tim Tams®, appeared on the front counter. "They're a good price," says Jan, and she began to rationalize their sale: "You know we don't have them *all the time*, and even OPAL don't say you can't *ever* eat chocolate biscuits: They just say they're a 'sometimes food'." Over the coming weeks more chocolates appeared, including South Australian sweet icons FruChocs®—apricot balls covered in milk chocolate. People were coming in just to ask about the chocolates—one very overweight man purchasing 13 blocks of chocolate (and meat pies). The proliferation of chocolate sales led one worker to wonder if the food bank had done the wrong thing. Another volunteer disagreed with her concerns: "But you've got to have something in here to attract the customers. And it sells well … if the boss wants me to make money." Tim Tams® appeared on the front counter next to the Dove® chocolates, purchased from a large warehouse food bank in Adelaide. We are told they are "just past their use by date but they taste just the same." We noticed these chocolates spreading around the shop, onto the "special" shelves for discounted items and also onto the main shelves. Chocolates available for Easter were quickly sold out.

Katie says: "We can make some money on the chocolate. Everyone likes chocolate and it gets sold quickly. Otherwise, our customers will just go elsewhere to get those things. Also, I think it is important for people to be able to afford something nice. They might be poor, they might be struggling and having a rough time of it, and if we can provide something that gives them a bit of a pleasure at a good price, well, what's wrong with that?"

A few weeks later Jan gets a phone call from her manager, the "boss," Susan White. When she gets off the phone she hurriedly announces: "Susan White is coming in. Hide the chocolate!" Vera grabs the blocks of chocolate from the counter and shoves them underneath the workbench before asking: "How about the Tim Tams®?" Jan thinks for a moment: "Put them under too, or ... wait [she hesitates], leave a packet up there on the counter ... that's alright. I mean it is a *sometimes* food." A local customer in the shop, who is puzzled as to why the chocolate has to be hidden, asks: "Aren't you allowed to sell chocolates in here? That's ridiculous! What do they think? That poor people can't have anything nice to eat?" "No, it's nothing like that," says Jan, "[i]t's because the food banks are meant to promote healthy eating, the focus on health, you know, everything in council is about health these days." The woman isn't convinced of the reasoning. "Don't all people have the right to choices? We are talking about adults here. I know that I eat quite healthily, but I like to have something nice, a bit of a treat too." Jan agrees, and adds: "We like to be able to provide something nice for the customers and at a good price, but well—it's just a tricky position that we're in."

When the OPAL program came into this community the staff were mindful of working in with local initiatives as part of building community capacity. But when OPAL staff came to work in the food banks tensions began to brew over the proposed changes. The tensions were around competing priorities: providing affordable and pleasurable foods versus providing "healthy" options. Food bank workers prioritized food affordability and choice over the sugar and salt content in food items.

The first day that Scarlette arrived in the food bank, Tanya wrote in her field notes that she looked "fresh and summery in a pristine short white skirt and white slim-fitted top. She looks out of place in the food bank, too clean, too crisp, too slim." She wanders around while she waits to speak to Jan, inspecting the meal packs and the items in the freezer, and then she walks behind the counter and sits herself at the table. Taking out a pen and notebook she explains why she has come to the food bank today: "We are about to launch our breakfast theme and we are interested in what you have here. We don't want to be doubling up on things you already do and we want to know if there are ways that we might be able to work together, that's if you're interested in that." Then she asks a series of questions: "I notice that you stock a lot of cereal here. What sorts of cereal do you tend to supply? When I spoke with staff at the other food bank they said they have to buy Coco Pops® and Nutrigrain® for the customers, that they are about choice and wanting to give the customers variety. Is that a priority here? What other breakfast foods do you have here? And dairy—what sorts of dairy items do you sell? Is the tinned fruit in juice or syrup? Do you ever sell frozen berries?" "Too expensive," says Jan. "Do you have dried fruit?" "Too expensive," says Jan.

The OPAL staff were soon known as the OPAL girls—young, female, and slim. They were tertiary-educated and full of enthusiasm for helping people to improve their eating habits, but, as one food bank worker reflected, they "are young pretty things without much experience." Food bank workers were aware of the embodied and classed demeanor of the nutritionists—well-intentioned but sometimes going a "bit too far" with the black and white rules around healthy eating. Workers in the food banks had lived and worked in the community for years and agreed that it was "hard for OPAL to understand what life is like for people here." One worker told us: "I've been a single mum on a pension and I've been poor. I remember having no money for simple things, like my own underwear. Now I was OK to go around without undies on, but I bet none of the OPAL girls have ever had an experience like that. So I guess it is hard for them to understand that most of the people here could not give a shit about the nutritional quality of their food."

One volunteer heard about the interview process for the new nutritionist and recounted her recollection of the applicants:

> *They were bright young things. One of them even had a PhD but you know people who have PhDs are, well not you, but they tend to be sort of posh, and in the interview it was like she was talking down to us! She was really toffee that one. The applicants were all well-groomed. You know, barbies and princesses. But that is not what we really need here is it? I mean they have to be able to relate to our customers and I just don't see how those girls could have those skills. I don't think they knew what they'd be in for working out here with the druggies in the northern suburbs.*

Some food banks workers wondered why a local person wasn't hired for the role: "I think they should put me in a nutritionist course and let me take on the role. … The people who come in here, do they come in to get food that is cheap and healthy? No. They just want food that is cheap.

They don't care about nutrition. I think OPAL is a great program and I really support it and I do love to work with them, but I don't know how much of a change families will make."

While OPAL staff remained employed for the entirety of our fieldwork, other health and community development workers in council seemed to come and go. After a long search for a new nutritionist, Annabelle moved to Adelaide in 2013 and came to see the food banks for the first time and meet the local volunteers. Jan was quick to tell Annabelle what she described as "the facts": "Look Annabelle, I'm going to tell you how it is … you'll notice that many of the things we stock here are not healthy, they are not OPAL-approved. But customers are on tight budgets and we like them to have the opportunity to buy things they might not be ordinarily able to afford. We try to offer people choice."

The concept of choice, as we noted in Chap. 2, is a "core concept informing contemporary policies on food and health" (Brooks et al. 2013). In an analysis of food and nutrition policy documents in the UK (1976–2010), Brooks et al. identify several frames of choice, including choice as personal responsibility (the duty to choose well), a problem (poor or wrong choices), an instrument for change (as in behavior change or nudging), and as freedom (choice as sovereign) (2013, pp. 153–155). Choice is often positioned in hegemonic power relations, and as a technology of self in which the neoliberal subject engages in self-care. We found that choice was also mobilized as a strategy of resistance to the diminishment of choice that OPAL presented, taking away people's rights and freedoms to eat what they wanted. Katie summed up this embodiment of choice as resistance:

> *You can tell all of these parents what foods to eat and what to avoid but they tend to already know these things and if you tell people what and how to eat they might get annoyed because you're thinking, "Mind your own business" and "I can eat what I like thank you very much." [A]nd we are talking about adults. They have the right to make their own decisions.*

This stance leverages the frame of freedom that choice operates with and uses it to counter the disciplining power of domination in healthy eating discourses.

Everyday Resistance, Choice, and Agency

As well as hiding stashes of chocolates under the counter, other small resistances were at play in the food banks. When OPAL devised salt- and sugar-free vegetable frittatas and vegetable muffins and trialed them as part of their breakfast initiative, with a view to forming new breakfast packs, food bank staff and local community members who tasted them were of the opinion that these items lacked flavor. A food bank coordinator explained the conundrum:

> *OPAL sent the recipe through. I don't know what they will be like. They are vegetarian muffins with zucchini—personally I don't like zucchini. Some of the OPAL stuff is a bit rough but I thought our baker June could make some up and we could see what they are like beforehand. I'd prefer sweet ones myself.*

The muffins also contained capsicum, carrot, corn, cheese, dried parsley, and chives. Picking up the glossy OPAL recipe card Angela says: "The people here are never going to cook that—they'd sooner chuck any leftover veg in the bin than use it for baking." When they are cooked, people say: "Vegetables don't belong in muffins … they could do with some salt." June agrees. "They are a bit bland. They are OK, but I don't think much of them." "Wouldn't buy one," Jan adds, "[t]hey are not really muffins, are they? I like sweet muffins but I don't know about these. Let's put them out the front of the shop to give away to the customers." Most customers do not take one when offered, and nobody who does take one comments favorably on their taste. To get around this problem food bank customers and staff perform their resistance to OPAL health promotion not only by maintaining their distinct taste preferences but also by secretly adding salty ingredients to the OPAL recipes they are cooking and promoting. Bemoaning the taste of OPAL vegetable frittatas, a worker told us "it really needs some salt but I know we can't put salt in it. I made this the other week and all of the volunteers agreed that it wasn't tasty, that it was missing something. Today I'm going to include some parmesan cheese." By stealthily "adding the salt" the food co-op workers found ways to maneuver their way around OPAL guidelines and make food more appetizing to local tastes.

These rejections of the ideals of healthy eating, self-discipline, and governance "demonstrate that people don't simply fall into line, and that possibilities for resistance are embedded in the multiplicity and dynamism of the relations that constitute power" (Warin 2011, p. 35). Social scientists have long reflected on how the limited agency of subordinate classes to mobilize and upset social hierarchies can facilitate the proliferation of small-scale acts of resistance (de Certeau 1984; Scott 1985/2008) and the regaining of symbolic power (Bourdieu 1984).

A similar but far more public performance of resistance was demonstrated by mothers in the English town of Rotherham (see Chap. 4) who were vilified for handing junk food to their children through the school gates at lunch time in defiance of Jamie Oliver's healthy school dinners (c.f. Fox and Smith 2011; Warin 2011). This was not what Jamie Oliver intended when he coined his "Pass it on" strategy in the Ministry of Food campaign! Once instructed in healthy eating and cooking, people were meant to pass on healthy recipes, not pass "junk" food literally on!

Rather than view these women's actions or indeed those in the food banks as a negative reactive to oppressive power (which resonates with narrow and dualist interpretations of Foucault's approach to resistance), we suggest that people are responding to the identity of "failure" that neoliberal governance entraps them in. The women of Rotherham rejected the subject position of inept mothers who couldn't be allowed to feed their own children. Local people in Playford also contested OPAL's expert positioning and tried to reinstate their own autonomy, freedom, and identities. These resistances are thus not a negation of power or a tactical reversal, but a generative "counter power" (Foucault 1979, pp. 218–220), in which local people challenge and subvert dominant discourses, and in doing so, attempt to position themselves in new ways.

In their own tactics of resistance against the "government of the girth" (Coveney 2014), food bank workers were also voicing the nuanced details of people's lives: Looking at the healthy OPAL breakfast packs Katie repeatedly says: "[T]his won't sell." With each pack containing two Weet-Bix (Australian cereal biscuits), a small serving of skim milk, and a tin of fruit in natural juices, it is unsweetened and unappealing to local tastes. Anticipating poor sales Angela bought the milk with the longest shelf life: "I can tell that they are just going to be sitting in the shop for months." For Katie it did not make sense that local families "who are already struggling financially" would spend the $2 on a single (and unsatiating) serve of the unpalatable pack. Like other food bank workers, Katie firmly believed that OPAL and the nutritionists had little understanding about the day-to-day lives of local people, who embody a history of working class pride, and disadvantage. Katie's criticism was that OPAL didn't understand the constraints under which people lived, and that OPAL was perceived as limiting choices, thus taking away people's freedom and agency. Moreover, the food bank was more than a place to purchase food; it provided a network of relationships for local people—"we're like a big family"—and workers were unhappy about the diminution of these important, sweetening relations.

* * *

Reducing one's sugar intake is not as straightforward as OPAL workers may have thought. Yates-Doerr points to the importance of tackling what we take for granted:

> *While the metabolic operations of nutrition may appear self-evident to those raised in a post-Cartesian era, where mechanistic explanatory structures are commonplace* (Coveney 2006), *the logic of nutrition in fact depends upon historically and culturally contingent understandings of food, bodies and life itself.* (2012, p. 298)

It is in relation to this daily grind of disadvantage that some families living in Playford posed a challenge to public health conceptualizations of sugar as mere "empty calories" and sought to reclaim the meanings of sweetness in their local worlds. We have argued elsewhere that the disciplining of bodies through careful eating in order to mitigate future risk does not necessarily have relevance for people who find it difficult to imagine a future beyond the next day or welfare payment (Warin et al. 2015). When horizons are shortened, sugary foods can sweeten moments of discomfort and provide an accessible way to "tinker" (Mol et al. 2010b, p. 13) with one's body and emotions through sensory gratification and enacting care roles for oneself and others.

Our findings suggest that it is essential to consider how social disadvantage creates conceptualizations of eating and care that are different from public health admonitions, and that sweetening difficult circumstances is important to pleasure, place, and social relations. When food is one of the few spaces of controllable, reliable pleasures people have, and they are being told that they can no longer purchase it or that they can no longer eat it, forms of resistance and resentment appear. Moreover, food pleasures are woven into acts of caring, part of coping with the tedium of economic woes and the daily necessities of (a lack of paid) work, family, and relationships (Bissell et al. 2016, p. 20).

Notes

1. Maccas is Australian slang for McDonalds®.
2. https://www.smh.com.au/business/consumer-affairs/australias-sugar-intake-described-by-experts-as-alarming-20160321-gnncw5.html
3. In her research on cancer survivorship, Kinshella (2017) notes how sugar is described by her participants as "a fuel" that "feeds" cancer:

   Sugar is not just bad, it is evil. It is malevolent and subverts the body's defense systems. It is devious and hides in other types of foods. It is sinfully sweet and seductive but once allowed into the body, it can feed destructive, uncontrollable growth. Participants talked about sugar as something cancer survivors have to be especially vigilant against.

4. A 2011 research paper, "The Australian paradox," written by dietitian Alan Barclay and nutritionist Jennie Brand-Miller, found a negative relationship between Australian obesity and sugar consumption (Barclay and Brand-Miller 2011). In their paper they claimed that sugar intake had actually declined in Australia and that sugar was not to blame for the rise in obesity and diabetes. Following media scrutiny (including claims of conflict of interest), the paper was discredited and shown to rely on incomplete data (Rikkers et al. 2013), as it excluded sugar contained in imported processed foods. An independent inquiry and a more recent paper by the authors in question refute these detractions and support their original argument (Brand-Miller and Barclay 2017).
5. Lollies is the name that Australians give to sugary confectionary (candy in the USA and sweets in the UK).
6. "Smoko" is an Australian slang term used to describe a short cigarette break.
7. Minties are a soft, chewable mint-flavored sweet.

References

Albon, D. (2005). Approaches to the study of children and sweet eating: A review of the literature. *Early Child Development and Care, 175*(5), 407–417.

Atwell, B. L. (2013). Is sugar the new tobacco: How to regulate toxic foods. *Annals Health L, 22*, 138.

Australian Bureau of Statistics. (2016). *Australian Health Survey: Consumption of added sugars, 2011–2012.* Retrieved from http://www.abs.gov.au/ausstats/abs@.nsf/Lookup/by%20Subject/4364.0.55.011~2011-12~Main%20Features~Added%20Sugars%20and%20Free%20Sugars~7

Barclay, A. W., & Brand-Miller, J. (2011). The Australian paradox: A substantial decline in sugars intake over the same timeframe that overweight and obesity have increased. *Nutrients, 3*(4), 491–504.

Barnes, M. (2012). *Care in everyday life: An ethic of care in practice.* Bristol: Policy Press.

Berlant, L. (2011). *Cruel optimism.* London: Duke University Press.

Bissell, P., Peacock, M., Blackburn, J., & Smith, C. (2016). The discordant pleasures of everyday eating: Reflections on the social gradient in obesity under neo-liberalism. *Social Science & Medicine, 159*, 14–21.

Borland, R., & Balmford, J. (2003). Understanding how mass media campaigns impact on smokers. *Tobacco Control, 12*(2), 45–52.

Bourdieu, P. (1984). *Distinction: A social critique of the judgment of taste* (trans: Nice, R.). Cambridge, MA: Harvard University Press.

Brand-Miller, J. C., & Barclay, A. W. (2017). Declining consumption of added sugars and sugar-sweetened beverages in Australia: A challenge for obesity prevention, *The American Journal of Clinical Nutrition, 105*(4), 854–863.

Brookes, G., & Harvey, K. (2015). Peddling a semiotics of fear: A critical examination of scare tactics and commercial strategies in public health promotion. *Social Semiotics, 25*(1), 57–80.

Brooks, S. D., Burges Watson, A., Draper, M., Goodman, H., Kvalvaag, H., & Wills, W. (2013). Chewing on choice. In E. J. Abbots & A. Lavis (Eds.), *Why we eat, how we eat: Contemporary encounters between foods and bodies* (pp. 149–169). Farnham: Ashgate.

Colchero, M. A., Rivera-Dommarco, J., Popkin, B. M., & Ng, S. W. (2017). In Mexico, evidence of sustained consumer response two years after implementing a sugar-sweetened beverage tax. *Health Affairs, 36*(3), 564–571.

Coveney, J. (2006). *Food, morals and meaning: The pleasure and anxiety of eating* (2nd ed.). London: Routledge.

Coveney, J. (2014). The government of girth. *Health Sociology Review, 17*(2), 199–213.

Cowan, J. K. (1991). Going out for coffee?: Contesting the grounds of gendered pleasures in everyday sociability. In P. Loizos & E. Papataxiarchēs (Eds.), *Contested identities: gender and kinship in modern Greece* (pp. 180–202). Princeton: Princeton University Press.

de Certeau, M. (1984). *The practice of everyday life.* Berkeley: University of California Press.

Dufty, W. (1975). *Sugar blues.* New York: Warner Books.

Fischler, C. (1987). Attitudes towards sugar and sweetness in historical and social perspective. In J. Dobbing (Ed.), *Sweetness* (pp. 83–98). Berlin: Springer.

Foucault, M. (1979). *Discipline and punish: The birth of the prison.* New York: Vintage Books.

Fox, R., & Smith, G. (2011). Sinner ladies and the gospel of good taste: Geographies of food, class and care. *Health & Place, 17*(2), 403–412.

Gillespie, D. (2008). *Sweet poison: Why sugar is making us fat.* Surry Hills: Penguin Group Australia.

Graham, H. (1994). Gender and class as dimensions of smoking behavior in Britain: Insights from a survey of mothers. *Social Science and Medicine, 38*(5), 691–698.

Harris, J. L., Pomeranz, J. L., Lobstein, T., & Brownell, K. D. (2009). A crisis in the marketplace: How food marketing contributes to childhood obesity and what can be done. *Annual Review of Public Health, 30*, 211–225.

Hastings, G., Stead, M., & Webb, J. (2004). Fear appeals in social marketing: Strategic and ethical reasons for concern. *Psychology & Marketing, 21*(11), 961–986.

Held, V. (2006). *The ethics of care: Personal, political, and global*. Oxford: Oxford University Press.

Hill, D. S., Chapman, B., & Donovanc, R. (1998). The return of scare tactics. *Tobacco Control, 7*(1), 5–8.

Holtzman, J. (2016). To love sugar one does not have to eat it. *Gastronomica: The Journal of Critical Food Studies, 16*(3), 44–55.

Joyce, B. (2017, February 17). Federal sugar tax proposals divide experts and federal government. *Sydney Morning Herald*. Retrieved from https://www.smh.com.au/politics/federal/sugar-tax-proposals-divide-experts-and-federal-government-20170217-guf0sd.html0

Kinshella, M. L. W. (2017). Quinoa buffets and sugar devils: Experiences of cancer survivorship through food. *Anthropology of Food* (12). Retrieved from https://journals.openedition.org/aof/8247

Lei, L., Rangan, A., Flood, V. M., & Louie, J. C. Y. (2016). Dietary intake and food sources of added sugar in the Australian population. *British Journal of Nutrition, 115*(5), 868–877.

Lim, D. C. (2013). Sugar, not fat, is the culprit. *British Medical Journal, 347*(2013). https://doi.org/10.1136/bmj.f6846.

Lupton, D. (2013). *Moral threats and dangerous desires: AIDS in the news media*. London: Routledge.

Lustig, R. (2013a, August 8). Toxic sugar. [ABC television series: *Catalyst*]. http://www.abc.net.au/catalyst/stories/3821440.htm

Lustig, R. (2013b). *Fat chance: The hidden truth about sugar, obesity and disease*. New York: Penguin.

McLennan, A. K., Ulijaszek, S. J., & Eli, K. (2014). Social aspects of dietary sugars. In L. Tappy, K. A. Lê, & M. I. Goran (Eds.), *Dietary sugars and health* (pp. 1–10). London: CRC Press.

Mintz, S. (1986). *Sweetness and power*. New York: Penguin.

Mol, A. (2008). *The logic of care: Health and the problem of patient choice*. London: Routledge.

Mol, A. (2010). Care and its values: Good food in the nursing home. In A. Mol et al. (Eds.), *Care in practice: On tinkering in clinics, homes and farms* (pp. 215–234). New London: Transaction Publishers.

Mol, A., Moser, I., & Pols, J. (2010a). *Care in practice: On tinkering in clinics, homes and farms*. New London: Transaction Publishers.
Mol, A., Moser, I., & Pols, J. (2010b). Care: Putting practice into theory. In A. Mol et al. (Eds.), *Care in practice: On tinkering in clinics, homes and farms* (pp. 7–26). New London: Transaction Publishers.
Nestle, M. (2016). Food industry funding of nutrition research: The relevance of history for current debates. *JAMA Internal Medicine, 176*(11), 1685–1686.
Pampel, F. C. (2012). Does reading keep you thin? Leisure activities, cultural tastes and body weight in comparative perspective. *Sociology of Health & Illness, 34*(3), 396–411.
Popkin, B. M. (2001). The nutrition transition and obesity in the developing world. *The Journal of Nutrition, 131*(3), 871S–873S.
Rikkers, W., Lawrence, D., Hafekost, K., Mitrou, F., & Zubrick, S. R. (2013). Trends in sugar supply and consumption in Australia: Is there an Australian paradox. *BMC Public Health, 13*(1), 668.
Rothman, A. J., Bartels, R. D., Wlaschin, J., & Salovey, P. (2006). The strategic use of gain- and loss-framed messages to promote healthy behavior: How theory can inform practice. *Journal of Communication, 56*(S1), S202–S220.
Scott, J. C. (1985/2008). *Weapons of the weak: Everyday forms of peasant resistance*. New Haven & London: Yale University Press.
Serematakis, C. (1994). *The senses still: Perception and memory as material culture in modernity*. Boulder: Westview Press.
Stoller, P. (1989). *The taste of ethnographic things*. Philadelphia: University of Pennsylvania Press.
Tronto, J. (1993). *Moral boundaries: A political argument for an ethic of care*. London: Routledge.
Warin, M. (2011). Foucault's progeny: Jamie Oliver and the art of governing obesity. *Social Theory & Health, 9*(1), 24–40.
Warin, M., & Dennis, S. (2005). Threads of memory: Reproducing the cypress tree through sensual consumption. *Journal of Intercultural Studies, 26*(1–2), 159–170.
Warin, M., Zivkovic, T., Moore, V., Ward, P. R., & Jones, M. (2015). Short horizons and obesity futures: Disjunctures between public health interventions and everyday temporalities. *Social Science & Medicine, 128*, 309–315.
World Health Organization. (2017). *Taxes on sugary drinks: Why do it?* Retrieved from http://apps.who.int/iris/bitstream/handle/10665/260253/WHO-NMH-PND-16.5Rev.1-eng.pdf;jsessionid=EDD383B6C4250C39F1946CC0403A1D3F?sequence=1
Yates-Doerr, E. (2012). The opacity of reduction: Nutritional black-boxing and the meanings of nourishment. *Food, Culture & Society, 15*(2), 293–313.
Zivkovic, T., Warin, M., Moore, V., Ward, P., & Jones, M. (2015). The sweetness of care: Biographies, bodies and place. In E. Abbotts, A. Lavis, & L. Attala (Eds.), *Careful eating: Bodies, food and care* (pp. 109–112). Farnham: Ashgate.

CHAPTER 6

Fat Can "Do Stuff"

We should have twigged earlier. At a statewide Obesity Prevention and Lifestyle (OPAL) training day early on in our fieldwork the social marketing team reflected on a presentation given by an invited academic. Simone, a public health sociologist with expertise in obesity studies, had suggested that the "lived experiences of fat people need to be involved in the development of obesity prevention programs" and that "positive portrayals of fat people in the social marketing material is important to engage the audience." The day following Simone's talk, two OPAL social marketers, Kellie and Mary, asked the group how they felt about use of the word "fat" as this was the word that Simone had used in her talk. The general response was that they found the word offensive. They were more comfortable with the words "obesity" or "overweight" because, as they explained, these are the "proper," clinical terms. Unbeknownst to the group, Simone had preferred to use the word "fat" because her Australian research with people who were overweight and obese and who had experienced significant stigma as a result found that the majority (80%) "hated or disliked the word obesity and would rather be called fat or overweight."

This exchange took on much more importance further down the track when we presented our findings about how research participants understood fatness. We didn't follow the taken-for-granted and dominant understanding of obesity. Like Simone we used the word fat rather than obese, we wrote about the value of fat and of being fat, as well as the more

M. Warin, T. Zivkovic, *Fatness, Obesity, and Disadvantage in the Australian Suburbs*,
https://doi.org/10.1007/978-3-030-01009-6_6

negative tropes that circulated in the community. Our multiple findings around fatness and the presentation of vernacular language around fatness proved to be the most controversial aspect of our research with our research partners. Our use of the word fat, and the positive aspects of being fat, jarred against the whole *raison d'être* of OPAL.

As discussed in Chap. 4, OPAL operated within a dominant biomedical framework that constructed obesity as an individual risk to health that required biopolitical regulation and containment—obesity and fatness were *only* a negative phenomenon. If fatness is only understood as negative, as a health risk, and as a stigmatized position, then there is no space to explore the complexity of large bodies or the pleasures of fatty foods. Just as they were aware of the harms of smoking, participants were fully aware of the oft-cited dangers of eating too much fat, sugar, and salt. They were cognizant that being "too big" could put them at risk for diabetes and other conditions. Being fat was sometimes experienced as a hindrance, as it made it harder to get to places, to walk, or to "show up" at your ex-husband's new wife at their wedding. Fat is, however, an ambiguous substance (Forth and Leitch 2014; Warin 2010), as it was also said to enhance well-being and was used as a material resource that acted to safeguard or augment bodily survival. Fat bodies worked to protect people, to fall back on as a store when times were really tough and there was no food in the cupboards, and to be a form of sexualized and gendered resourcefulness (Zivkovic et al. 2018).

Our findings align with many historical and cross-cultural studies that point to the socially and aesthetically desirable qualities of fat (Becker 1995; Pollock 1995; Popenoe 2004; Powdermaker 1960; Renzaho 2004; Sobo 1993, 1997; Yates-Doerr 2015). In her ethnographic work in Jamaica, Elisa Sobo (1993, 1997) found that robust bodies and appetites were valued as attractive, sociable, and sexually "ripe." "People tied to a network of kin," writes Sobo (1997, p. 256), "are always plump." Jamaicans meet social obligations to share with and nurture kin through food. Anthropologist Rebecca Popenoe (2004), in her work with Moor women in Niger, attended to a cultural aesthetic of female corpulence as "good, beautiful, and desirable" (2004, p. 188). Moor practices of fattening oneself (and the bodies one cares for) create a socially embedded body with "meaty flesh [which] is the paragon of sexual attractiveness" (2004, p. 189). Similarly, anthropologist Emily Yates-Doerr's work on obesity in Guatemala highlights how fatness (for oneself and for others one cares for) can be attractive and a sign of health and happiness (2015, p. 176).

As described in Chap. 2, the fat acceptance, fat activism, and Health at Every Size (HAES) movement strongly reject dominant discourses that accept the associations between fat, disgust, and ill-health (Aphramor 2005; Solovay and Rothblum 2009). In promoting a fat-positive approach to large bodies, fat activists present large bodies as beautiful and "flabulous" (Wann 1998). The range of fat activists and fat studies scholars is diverse, but these groups share a common goal to highlight positive experiences of fat embodiment (Colls 2012; Monaghan 2005) and to celebrate large bodies as attractive, agentive, powerful, and positive (Pausé 2017).[1]

Fat, however, in public health and medical fields has been forced into what Land refers to as "a parasitic union with obesity" (Land 2018, p. 77). Fat, she continues, has become "consumed by a pervasive and potent obesity apparatus—a carefully curated assemblage that is profoundly complicit in, and generative of, neoliberal systems of governmentality" (Land 2018, p. 77). In this apparatus of fat knowledge, fat is always constructed as an unsightly health risk (Lupton 2013). Our research partners were deeply invested in this singular view of fat as a health risk.

Representing fat as positive or productive—even using the word "fat" and writing or talking about other euphemisms or joking phrases that participants used to spar with each other (such as "thunder thighs," "whale," "big bums," or "big shapely arses") was viewed by our local and state government partners as taboo. Cross-cultural work, however, demonstrates that calling someone fat "is not ordinarily an insult" (Hardin 2015, p. 178), and can be used to illustrate the ambivalence about the meanings of fat. While we wanted to explore the ways in which the language of fat was strategically used, through humor and sexuality, to distance the stigma of obesity shaming, our research partners asked us to remove quotes that they understood as simply reproducing (rather than counteracting) stigma. While we wanted to think about fat as enacted in lives that had little [economic] fat to cut, we were asked to find more "palatable" and less "classed" contexts in which to talk about fat.

In this chapter we explore the socio-materiality of bodies and practices; how people experienced, enacted, and embodied fat as positive and productive or disabling in their day-to-day practices in the Australian suburbs. Importantly, this is not to suggest that the participants in our study were immune to dominant representations of fat as an unhealthy trope. While participants did not distinguish between the nutritional categories of "bad fats" (saturated fat and trans fat) and "good fats" (monounsaturated, polyunsaturated, and omega-3 fatty acids), they expressed knowledge of fat as both something inside the body (body fat) and as something outside the body (fatty food) that is unhealthy and can lead to a range of health complications. As Jan, a 53-year-old mother and grandmother, asserted, "[o]bviously if you're fatter you're prone to heart disease, stroke, diabetes, I mean you're just a walking time bomb aren't you? So yeah, it [fat] does matter" (Zivkovic et al. 2018). During the course of our fieldwork Jan said she would never get on any scales as she didn't want to know her weight and was not interested in attending to it. More than 12 months later, when we saw her on the day of the royal visit (Prince William and Kate came to Elizabeth in April 2014), she stood tall and moved her hands along the edges of her changed figure. "I've lost 17 kilos" she said, beaming with pride. Moments later she explained: "I had to do it for my heart. I want to live." Fat had multiple registers, and participants could hold polyvalences of fat, depending on the context.

In exploring fat we attended both to what people, our participants, did to or with their bodies *and* to what it was that their bodies, and their fat, did to them. We extend the recent writings on the culture and materiality of fat (Forth and Leitch 2014; Warin 2015), attending to what Colls calls "the materializations of fatness" (Colls 2007, p. 353). In this move toward materialities, the social *and* material life of fat is repositioned "not as mutually exclusive," but in "constant interplay and connectedness" (Warin 2015; c.f. Hardin 2015). In the lives of our participants the presence of fat on their own bodies and on the bodies of others drew a variety of responses that provided an ethnographic grounding that located the substance of fat in new ontological terrains.

Attending to the enactments of fat is to take seriously its materiality in order to release it from the grip of representation that constricts bodies to singular, simpler dimensions that Probyn (2008, p. 402) describes as "extraordinarily thin." We thus flesh out fat as a complex "assemblage in which persons *and* fats are participants" (Bennett 2010, p. 42, [emphasis added]). By anthropomorphizing fat and according it a degree of agency, Bennett makes space to accommodate "the strivings and trajectories of fats as they weaken or enhance the power of human will, habits, and ideas" (2010, p. 43). Providing ethnographic examples of what fat does, how it ebbs and flows, labors, and performs power in the day-to-day lives and bodies of research participants, we foreground its agency "to exert forces and create effects" (Bennett 2007, p. 133).

The Fullness of Fat

There were many instances in our fieldwork when the fullness of fat was described as a form of generosity, or authenticity, and in terms of warming and nurturing both bodies and relationships. On her last day of working in one of the food banks, with three other volunteers, Tanya wrote in her field notes about how hot it was:

> *The forecast is 31 degrees [88 fahrenheit] today, creeping up to 40 on Thursday. But inside the shop the air conditioner blasts and I feel chilled to the bone. When I look cold Jan shakes her head. "No bloody meat on ya, Tanya—That's your problem. Not like me. I come with plenty of insulation." Later when I comment on my love of summer and hot balmy nights and my dislike of winter, Jan again mentions our differing amounts of body fat. "Well you wouldn't like summer so much if you were inside my body. It's pretty bloody hot in here, there's a lot more to carry around. Give me winter any day."*

This need for more body warmth in colder weather reminded us of the more nuanced account of fat presented by Throsby (2015) in her investigation of marathon swimming. Throsby introduces the concept of "heroic fat" to problematize the "normative opposition of 'fit' and 'fat'" (2015, p. 771), which come together in swimmers' purposeful gaining of fat as an undesirable but "necessary act of bodily discipline and sacrifice" (for buoyancy and insulation). Granted social capital through their status as athletes, Throsby demonstrates how athletes "endure" and "overcome" fatness, embodying a self-sacrifice that "immunizes the heroically fat swimmer against the negative stigma of 'real' fatness" (Throsby 2015, p. 772). This fatness, she suggests, and the ways in which swimmers slap, jiggle, and wobble their own and each other's fat, is used to create a "much more complicated and contradictory mix of acceptance, celebration and fat phobia" (Throsby 2013).

Shoppers who came into the food bank did not have the luxury of such "heroic status" ascribed to their bodies. They were being asked to reduce their body sizes through dietary changes, and many disliked the tenor of moral judgment that accompanied such lifestyle changes. This was most evident in OPAL's stated preference for "reduced-fat" over "full-fat" products. Katherine, an English migrant, didn't agree with the changes she saw on the food bank shelves and in the fridges. She recalled how when she was young she'd "get a quart of milk with a thick glob of fat on top." "There," she said "was your calcium and your protein that would really keep you going to lunch. That's how you really look after kids so that they can concentrate at school. There is nothing like that here." Contained in this full-fat milk was the goodness of fat, a substance that provided sustenance and feelings of fullness. These positive attributions of fat are similar to some (not all) of the nutritionist views that Yates-Doerr (2015) writes about in her research, where fat was sometimes emphasized as a "healthy part of food" because "the body needs fat" (2015, p. 182).

Volunteers in the food bank sometimes cringed at the thought of reducing fats, as they viewed this as a stripping away of nutrition, pleasure, and personal choice. In one conversation prior to an OPAL planning day, Helen reminded the other volunteers that they'd have to take their own lunch as only scones would be provided. Katie chipped in: "If OPAL are organizing the scones there will probably be no butter. I went to something the other day and OPAL had scones without any butter." Helen shook her head incredulously. "Scones without butter? Aren't you all adults? Are you now incapable of making up your own mind as to whether or not you are going to eat butter? I think adults should have a choice." "I couldn't agree with you more, Helen" said Katie in support.

In many ways, the disgruntlement about having to reduce or eliminate fat in diets stood as a sign of much broader tensions around what it meant to "cut the fat." Often it was the foods that were deemed to be healthier, such as skim milk or bacon with no visible fat, that were viewed as less satisfying, and also more expensive. Food bank workers became exasperated when their efforts to accommodate the price of foods were dismissed in favor of statements that prioritized health, and tensions began to appear. People raised their eyebrows with incredulity when OPAL staff said everyday items like Cornflakes®, fruit pieces in syrup, and full-cream milk were "not healthy." Volunteers began to clench their teeth in frustration: "Look, we're not nutritionalists [sic], we're just trying to do our job, but there you have it—no Cornflakes®. And on top of that the fruit is no good either. Well *really* fruit! Apparently fruit's not healthy! We're not doing well are we?"

Full-fat and skim milk was a constant flash point in the food bank. The OPAL rule that all children over the age of two should drink reduced-fat milk was rejected outright by some community members who believed that in consuming low-fat milk children were "not getting enough nutrition." Skim milk was placed in breakfast packs made up in the food bank for children. Like Katherine, Katie also wanted local children to have full-fat milk and told us how she had persuaded Amelia (an OPAL worker) to change this. "I told her that since we are doing these [breakfast packs] for the school, and since they are specifically for kids who are not eating well at home, that it was important for them to have their full-cream milk rather than skim," said Katie with a bit of a giggle. "And she said 'OK' Amelia did. So there you go, it is just a game of words. You have to know the right things to say to them and then they'll let you get away with anything."

But sometimes this tactic of persuasion did not work so well. It was well known that some of the food bank volunteers bristled when having to work with the OPAL staff. One role in the food bank was to take the mobile van out into the community and run courses and training sessions with children in schools. We were told that one food bank volunteer, Peta, "didn't get along with the OPAL girls very well ... in fact her and Amelia couldn't work together." The example used to demonstrate their difficult working relationship was about milk. "They went out to do a cooking demonstration together at a living skills center and were both entirely inflexible. Peta had brought along full-cream milk and Amelia wanted skim milk; she wouldn't use the full-cream milk and Peta wouldn't get the skim and so on—so there was a battle. There needs to be some flexibility on our side and on OPAL's as well. We need to be able to work together." This stand-off over full-fat and skim milk exemplified general resistance to being told what and how to eat, and a disdain not only for the "thinness" of skim milk, but for the perceived inflexibility of the health mantra.

There were other examples of working tensions that concerned people's body sizes. When council hired a nutritionist to work with OPAL and the food banks, we asked why a local volunteer, Leonie, might not have been considered. Jan was quick to support Leonie and explained:

> *People really like her but I think that council wouldn't want her doing this job because, well just because of her weight. She is very overweight and it is not the picture of health that they want to be promoting. And I sort of get where they are coming from but there are many large people out here and people mightn't be so quick to take on health advice from young, thin, pretty things. I know that I'm overweight too, let's face it, but if I were going to promote healthy eating among a group of people in the community I could say, "Look, I'm trying to lose weight too," and I think that would be OK, I mean people could then relate to me because we are in the same boat in terms of being big, you know?*

Being relatable meant "being real." Some food bank staff suggested that the OPAL girls "need to get real." Jan, for example, loved to have instant soups for lunch when she was working. "I love 'cup-a-soups'," she says, "they are my favorite." But Poppy told her they were "no good for her." "But they're not high in calories," retorted Jan, hoping this would please Poppy. The problem, Poppy said, was that "they have too much salt," Jan batted the conversation back, still trying to win: "Better than a meat pie though." "Hmm … not much better," replied Poppy.

Following that competitive exchange and a few days later, when Poppy was not around, Jan remained wedded to her stance: "But they *are* better than a meat pie, I reckon. And they are really yum and handy. I think the OPAL girls have got to get a bit real. I'm busy. I like something that is quick and still tastes good." Jan prioritizes taste and convenience, whereas Poppy prioritizes good nutrition. Jan continues to bolster her argument, making a case that cutting too much fat can be bad for your health: "If you ask me the OPAL girls are all looking really thin. Poppy is the thinnest she has ever been and I don't think she is looking that good, and Amelia has lost weight too. Amelia has lost it due to stress; she has just left a relationship. But the others, I think it's a worry that they are all that thin." Here, Jan makes an important distinction between different types of thinness. Thinness through stress is acceptable, but thinness through restricting foods "that are not good for you" is presented as "a worry." The food bank workers did not unequivocally align thinness with health; rather, thinness could be a sign of being unhealthy.

These valued concepts of fatness resonate with what Emily Yates-Doerr found in her Guatemalan fieldwork. For many of the women in her research, pleasure was found in fat, and fatness could be healthy (2015, p. 181). Fatness "pertained to an imponderable, innumerable richness that might loosely approximate happiness but which was more akin to fullness—the *rica* [delicious or tasty]—of satisfaction" (2015, p. 181). Like the contentment one might feel with a fat wallet, the Guatemalan women described feeling the content of fatness when surrounded by plentiful foods shared among kin. For them this represented abundance and to be or feel fat meant that life was going well (ibid.).

This conceptual difference between fatness and obesity is key, as this is not a cultural preference for obesity, but a cultural valuing of abundance, pleasure, and relationality. Obesity is a term discovered in measurement and weights, whereas fatness had much broader implications. Both can exist simultaneously.

Fuller Figures

When a nutritionist position was created in the council, we saw how people's relationships were tempered around body sizes and attitudes to foods that were not "OPAL-approved." Annabelle had applied for the nutritionist position from a country OPAL site in South Australia. She had already visited the food bank staff with "the boss," and it was noted that she was "all dressed up," which Jan said immediately created unease—"What have we got here?" But the day she arrived to start work in the food bank she looked tired and didn't embody the joviality or enthusiasm that often marked OPAL staff. "I've been up late packing so I'm not getting much sleep," she said apologetically as she yawned. Annabelle was moving to a new house in a local suburb in the City of Playford. The first thing we noticed about Annabelle was that she was tall and of medium build. She was not overly thin, which was another stark contrast from most other OPAL staff. As Katie took her around in an orientation to the shop, she said: "We sell some things in the shop to make a profit. We don't really make a profit out of our meal packs, but we do make some money from selling biscuits." Katie picked up one of the Kindy Packs of sweet biscuits and fruit drinks which contained sugar. "These are our Kindy Packs. Parents buy these for their children to take to school and they are very popular. For $1.40 they just walk out the door. I know they are not healthy and if we were doing them for some OPAL events they would have to contain water instead of juice and perhaps dried fruit instead of the chips or biscuits but the way they are here, now, they sell well."

Annabelle fumbled through the assortment of Kindy Packs on the counter and spotted one containing Shapes (a small savory biscuit). "Oh I love Shapes" she confessed. Katie looked pleased. "Oh you do? You like Shapes?" she repeated it as a question, smiling. "Yeah, I used to live on them. Really. When I was younger in my teens and early twenties. I'd have a packet a day. I'd eat them through the day and for lunch; they were a main part of my diet," said Annabelle. Katie looked shocked to hear such words come out of a nutritionist's mouth. "You ate them *every day*? When did you come to realize that wasn't such a good idea, that it wasn't very healthy?" "Oh it took me a while. It wasn't until I started doing some studies in physical education. I had a sort of health and fitness assessment as part of my training at the time. I was really overweight back then and so after the assessment it became quite clear to me that what I was eating was making me unhealthy and put on weight, and so I started to make some changes." Katie gazed at Annabelle approvingly.

> *I think it is very important that you have had the experience of being overweight. If you are someone who has been tiny all of your life, how are you going to understand what it is like to be big or what it is like to develop the habits that can lead a person to become big. I think for your position here it is very useful for you, if you are going to connect with some of the people who come in here who are very big and who do not always eat the healthy options, I think it is good that you have some direct personal experience of eating the unhealthy foods, of having a taste for them and of being large yourself.*

Annabelle's down-to-earth approach and her own experiences of being a larger body size signified that she was a "real person"—practical, and not a "barbie doll or princess." Annabelle was effectively food bank "approved"!

The coordinator at the other food bank was also pleased with Annabelle. Like Katie, she was wary of being told how to run things by an outsider, and wanted to be upfront with Annabelle and to lay down the law about how things were done in the food banks. While they were driving around in the mobile van, Jan took the opportunity to set things straight: "Look Annabelle, I'm gonna tell you how it is. On Fridays we get a lot of food come in from the [city] food bank. I order the food and there is a lot of shit. We get lots of biscuits and unhealthy foods because I order them. The customers like them. I like them and the volunteers here like them and I'm going to continue to order them." Jan told us that Annabelle was "totally cool" with this and said: "I'm not here to change you or the food banks in terms of getting rid of stuff. I am just going to work with what you've already got to see how we can make some improvements there. So that is fine. I am totally open to that." Jan reiterated the importance of allowing shoppers to have choice, and to respect people's choices, whatever they are. Taking a leaf out of neoliberal discourse, Jan upheld the view that "we are not going to nanny them and tell them what they should and shouldn't do." "Annabelle" she said, "agreed, so I think we are on the same page there."

Annabelle's relaxed approach to food and eating (and the clothes that she wore, such as "trackie-dacks"—Australian slang for tracksuit pants) was frequently contrasted with the style of OPAL staffers. She was described not only as "more real" but also "as more flexible" than the other OPAL girls. Food bank staff said that OPAL pushed the "healthy, healthy, healthy" mantra, whereas Annabelle presented as someone "who thinks that nutrition is not the main priority here, even though that is what council wants." As an example of her flexibility, Annabelle's approach to wine was presented as "more practical, and more real." Katie recounted the story of when Scarlette, an OPAL worker, talked to the food bank staff about the new healthy eating guidelines and how a glass of wine should be 100 ml, no more than that. Katie said to Tanya: "I can imagine both her and Amelia sticking to that, but I think Annabelle might be more balanced. She might be a bit more like you and me and have *a real glass.* I think the others might take it a bit too far."

An additional reason why the food bank workers liked Annabelle is that she positioned fatness not as an individual failure of willpower, but as an addiction. She suggested to the workers that a person who overeats and eats all the wrong salty and sugary processed foods is like someone who cannot stop smoking or drinking or taking drugs. Katie responded to this explanation, saying: "They are all addicts in a way and that kind of makes sense to me." The idea that highly palatable foods are addictive helped Katie understand the enjoyment of certain foods and the difficulty of "just stopping eating them." In addition, the idea that sugary and high-fat foods can disrupt parts of the neurological system that deal with self-control and pleasure can be rationalized as absolving responsibility for the common accusation of "poor behavior" and "poor choices" that is leveled at people who are obese. A more biologically determinist explanation, while still relying on individualist ideology, distances people from the shame and blame that accompanies stereotypes of obesity.

Framing obesity as an addiction, however, is a double-edged sword. Addiction is commonly constructed as a disease (Reinarman 2005), and a dominant framework for understanding illicit drug use or alcoholism. It has a discursive history, and "like obesity, addiction functions as a diagnostic and normalizing tool that attempts to institute conceptual borders in our tacit, unfixed knowledge of deviant bodies, to name pathology and thus arrest its development" (Murray 2008, p. 63). In a normalizing system, people can be subject to discipline—"for their own good"—as a consequence of such incapacity to care for themselves. Versions of this might be seen in punitive welfare policies for people identified as obese and in need of hard-line "incentives" to break addiction, such as linking certain food provision to welfare payments (as with the Basics Card in South Australia), making exercise a prerequisite for receiving welfare, or withholding sickness benefits for people who don't lose weight (as put forward in the UK by the Conservative government in 2015) (Lancet 2015).

No Room to "Cut the Fat"

In asking participants "how do people get fat?" we inadvertently prompted discussions of what fat does to their own bodies and to the bodies of others. There was a range of responses which represented the diverse explanations that people held about why people put on weight. While the "too much food and too little exercise" mantra could easily roll off people's tongues, their responses as to why people became fat were often much more nuanced and contextualized within life circumstances. We heard many agentive and positive accounts about fatness, unsettling ideas about fat as a passive or inert substance, and also diverging from negative portrayals of fat. Fat was rationalized as a form of self-preservation and survival; strengthening, protecting, and cushioning participants' bodies, literally and figuratively, from the hard knocks and exhaustion (Berlant 2010) of life.

When we asked participants about being large ("Does it matter if someone is a large body size? Do you worry about people you know that have a large body size?"), they often pushed back against the "problem" of obesity, subverting associations between fat and ill-health. Steve, an unemployed man in his 20s explained that his main concern with body size was "when you're nothing but bone. Shouldn't be like that because it only takes a slight push and then you're stuffed." As Yvette, a mother of two living on a disability pension, told us "carrying some extra weight" could safeguard against illness and hardship. Reactions to thinness or to fatness, as Nadine Ehlers (2014, p. 109) observes, depends on the contexts in which bodies are embedded. Poverty and social disadvantage may render fat "desirable," an asset, and not "surplus" or "waste" (Ehlers 2014, p. 109). Often it was thin bodies, rather than fat ones, that became sites of alarm. In the field, thinness carried a symbolic load and it was not a physical trait that participants unequivocally aspired to. On the contrary, thinness was often read as a sign of drug addiction and illness in the bodies of "speed freaks," "meth heads," and "anorexics," and it was encoded with messages about hardship and social disadvantage. Tove et al. (2006), in their comparative psychological study of UK and South African women, similarly found that in contexts of low socioeconomic status, thinness for the rural South African women was associated with perceptions of ill-health (Tove et al. 2006), as weight loss was a clear indication of infectious diseases, such as HIV/AIDS or parasitic diseases.

The striking lack of body fat on impoverished frames could provoke reactions of repulsion, and participants described these bodies as "looking ill" and "worn down." Angela, a middle-aged mother and grandmother, spoke to these cultural registers of thinness when she explained that she had lost a lot of weight. A poor sleeper, Angela relied on coffee, cigarettes, antidepressants, and sleeping pills, rather than meal times, to sequence her days. Tall and thin, she told us that she had struggled for years to keep any weight on. A long-drawn-out encounter with glandular fever alongside menopause progressed to chronic fatigue, exasperating depression, and triggering digestive ailments. Angela shed more kilos. Becoming increasingly gaunt, she felt anxious about the weight loss and told us that it made her look "haggard," "weak," and "aged." However, by the end of our project Angela acquired new fleshy layers, padding out her previously withered body and ironing out the wrinkled appearance that had "really scared" her. As with Wilson's analysis of the ways in which the alimentary tract, pills, and neurology cohabit, entwine, and annex each other as they "bind, braid, branch and cleave" (2015, p. 150), Angela demonstrates how the drugs she imbibed, her hormones, and her emotional states are all inherently shaped by one another.

The existential angst that arises in encounters with emaciation is described by Forth (2014) in his work on the culture and materiality of fat. "When contained within the bodily envelope greasy and sticky fat enhances the softness of soft tissues, fills in potentially unsightly concavities, and blunts the hard edges of bones" and its lack is "the most telling signs of the skeleton—an unpleasant reminder of human mortality" (Forth 2014, p. 62). Stripped of fat, bodies appear aged and in decline, which Forth suggests may be one reason that "varying degrees of plumpness have functioned in many cultures as evidence of health, youth and vitality" (2014, p. 62). Departing from disgust, disease, and a discourse of excess—the characteristics often associated with fat bodies—participants revealed that the storage of extra fat could act as "back up" in times of illness, producing a healthier and more youthful appearance.

Fat is a substance that shapes both the contour and function of bodies, and it makes a difference to everyday life. It is, as Mol suggests, "enacted" in practice (Mol 2002, p. 32), and for participants fat was enacted in "breathlessness," "sweating more," "bad knees," "bad backs," "bad hearts," and "additional hurdles" to overcome or to bend over in routine acts of daily living, like tying up shoelaces. However, these experiences of being fat exist alongside myriad other enactments.

Fat as Gendered Labor

A "mercurial and ambiguous" substance, body fat is conceived and experienced in a multitude of shifting and contradictory ways (Forth 2013, p. 135). Even in one body fat could elicit a variety of contradictory responses. Reminiscent of Edmonds' (2010) study on "fat sculpting" in Brazil, where fat is removed from one location and injected into buttocks and breasts, fleshy bulges on some bodily sites were coveted and held greater aesthetic and sexual appeal than other body parts. Participants described how "a big shapely arse" or "big boobs" could compensate for "thunder thighs" or a "mummy tummy." In the words of Maggie, a 28-year-old mother, "[s]o as long as my boobs stick out more than my belly it's all sweet."

Candy, a gregarious single mum, vividly illustrated the value of different kinds of fat. At the commencement of our study Candy was proud that she had reduced her weight by "eating less" and exercising "a little bit." But there were body parts that she would prefer to augment rather than diminish. Pushing up her small breasts with her hands, she declared woefully: "I have lost my girls since I lost my weight." Unlike her mother with "massive norks" much coveted by Candy, she had not been large-breasted before the weight loss and mourned the flattened contours of her breasts—"the girls"—because, she told us, "they used to get me stuff" (Zivkovic et al. 2018).

Like many participants in this study, Candy lived on a government pension and spoke of being "poor." Supporting herself and her daughter on a tight budget left her with limited resources to go out or "to have fun." With a penchant for live music, Candy relished the opportunity to "go to a pub and see a band" or play eight-ball, steadfastly resisting the purchase of alcoholic drinks she could not afford on her limited income. In line with Ehlers' (2014) "labour of fat," this is the domain where Candy put her girls "to work." With pushed up cleavage over low-cut dresses, she performs to the male gaze over games of pool, explaining with pride that "they get me drinks," before listing "the girls'" other notable functions: "[T]hey get me off speeding fines and on bad hair days I can hoik [push] them out and no one notices [my hair]." A moment later she adds that "they can also feed babies"—a job that Candy found "too icky" (disgusting).

The gendered labor of Candy's body depended on her breast tissue, and the absence of this form of fat, as Ehlers notes in her work on breast reconstruction surgery, is "threatening or destabilising to gender identity"

(2014, p. 109). Toward the end of the project Candy was relieved that she'd put a few kilos back on, excitedly declaring: "Oh my girls! I got my girls back!" Delighted with their "return," she could once again put them to work, getting drinks and getting out of car fines in a material transaction that affords small pleasures and social mobility amid poverty and disadvantage.

Anthropologist Simone Dennis makes the same point in her phenomenological exploration of smoking and smoker's practices. In her Australian fieldwork she describes a female participant who uses cigarettes and the blowing of smoke from pursed lips to extend herself out into the world, to accentuate her attempts to "look sexy and elegant" as she smokes (2013, p. 288). Like the sexualized exercise of flesh in our fieldwork, the expulsion of smoke from her mouth was put to seductive labor. How it was expelled onto men ("around the side of his face, like a caress … or blown straight into their face, into their eyes") would signal flirtatious practice or clear unavailability (ibid.). For this smoking participant, and our participants who were large, fatness and smoking afforded pleasure and gendered desire in the immediacy of the present.

The matter of fat intersects materiality with social circumstances to create "multiple kinds of fat with different actions and behaviors" (Kendrick 2013, p. 250). "Thinking metabolically" about fat and food—what it becomes when it "descends into visceral depths … to become part of the body's biochemical hustle and flow, which includes the growth and decline of fat tissue" (2013, p. 237)—opens up possibilities of "multiple fatnesses" (2013, p. 250). The rise and fall of Candy's breasts draw attention to the activities of fatty tissues, clearly articulating how multiple fatnesses pervade bodies.

Fat as Power

We turn now to consider how fat operates as power in circumstances of physical and sexual abuse. The incidence of domestic violence assessments and child protection assessments within this area is more than double the incidence in metropolitan Adelaide (Government of South Australia 2010). Many of the women we spoke to frequently narrated traumatic and violent biographies and they had developed resourceful and resilient strategies, using the agency of fat to "get by" in their everyday lives. Alongside self-medication through cigarettes, drugs, and alcohol, women told us that they had cared for themselves through food. "Comfort eating" for

Jude, and others, was a way to find small moments of relief in difficult life circumstances. In eating sweet and fatty food, Jude reoriented her senses away from an abusive relationship, for which she now takes antidepressants to prevent the intrusion of memories, "flashbacks" to this terrifying past. "Motivated by stress, a desire for self-medication," eating, like taking drugs, can become "one of the few spaces of controllable, reliable pleasure people have" (Berlant 2011, p. 115). Indigenous participant Pearl, to whom this chapter will turn, also used the terminology of "self-medication" (re)conceptualizing fat as "powerful" material protection "against the many predators out there." Such strategies are common, as Roxane Gay reminds us in her recent book *Hunger*, in which she details the lifelong consequences of her decision to make her body as big as possible as a form of self-protection against the shame of being raped (2017):

> *My body was broken. I was broken … I was hollowed out. I was determined to fill the void, and food was what I used to build a shield around what little was left of me. I ate and ate and ate in the hopes that if I made myself big, my body would be safe. I buried the girl I was because she ran into all kinds of trouble. I tried to erase every memory of her, but she is still there, somewhere. She is still small and scared and ashamed.* (Gay 2017, p. 19)

Eating can be a practice of care in precarious lives (Zivkovic et al. 2015); however, eating is also a material and metabolic process connecting the outside with the insides of bodies (Kendrick 2013) and transforming them through the accumulation of additional adipose tissue. Or, as Bennett (2010, p. 40; emphasis added) explains, to eat food is to "enter into an assemblage" where "food *coacts* with the hand that places it in one's mouth, with the metabolic agencies of intestines, pancreas, kidneys, with cultural practices of physical exercise, and so on, food can generate new human tissues."

The substance of fat, therefore, is not only acted upon (by consuming bodies) but acts back upon the body in a sympathetic resonance (Bennett 2011), becoming, as Pearl's story shows, a physical defense that protects people from a hostile world. An elder for her Indigenous community, 55-year-old Pearl told us that she was "the sole survivor" of severe child abuse and had been born to "drinkers and druggers" in rural Queensland. Her siblings died in childhood from suicide, cancer, meningitis, and a pulmonary aspiration during a stress-induced catatonic state. Stooped over in a wheelchair, her misshapen legs cannot walk, and she relies on methadone to relax the pain and tensions her body has carried over a lifetime of physical and sexual abuse and regular acts of self-harm.

To keep "a barrier" between herself and the world, Pearl told us that she would "eat like she was starving" adding extra "bags" (rolls of fat) to insulate and guard her body. Reaching 109 kg, being fat was a strategy "to stop being hurt seriously" in her encounters with violent men. In contrast to Candy's breasts, Pearls bags acted to avert the male gaze by keeping men away. To be fat for Pearl was thus to be "powerful" because it protected and strengthened her body to counter-attack in a "series of potentialities" that "emerge both from and towards fat" (Colls 2007, p. 362).

While outside the scope of this book, a conversation with an eminent Australian anthropologist points to interesting questions about fat in Indigenous communities. Having years of experience with Indigenous communities in the remote areas of Cape York Peninsula and the Northern Territory, Peter Sutton recounted to us his own pleasurable experiences of eating turtle fat while field-working in these communities. A broader search of the literature identified the cultural significance of fat in Indigenous Australian communities, pointing both to its practical use and to its symbolic representations. Traditionally valued for its high calorific content, the consumption of animal fats is associated with stamina and strength, and the topical application of liquefied fat (oils and grease) triggers a glistening of the skin linked to beauty and sexual arousal (Devitt 1991; McDonald 2003). Fat is also a spiritually powerful substance, containing the vital forces of the ancestors and of life (Redmond 2001, p. 133; pers. comm. Peter Sutton). Of course, the heterogeneity of Indigenous Australians would mean a similar heterogeneity of fat, but the value of such cross-cultural understandings is that they point to the multiple practices and meanings of fat.

* * *

Earlier on in this chapter we acknowledged the excellent ethnographic work that describes the ways in which fulsome bodies are often given high status and value. This work is taken up by popular discourses in very particular ways—perhaps exemplified by Jessica Simpson's reality TV show where she visited "fattening huts" in Uganda (http://www.youtube.com/watch?v=wem6aHYNeRU). Upon learning about the process of fattening brides, she exclaimed: "This is the complete opposite of everything I have ever known." Jessica is astonished that the hut is lined with "gourd after gourd of cow's milk" that the bride-to-be drinks from. The fact that fatness is here constructed as a desirable and positive attribute, rather than negative, is what surprises Jessica. The show draws on classic Eurocentric concepts in which a positive and negative dichotomy is applied to fatness. Made for the consumption of Western viewers, the show positions the Ugandan villagers as ignorant about the perils of obesity, as in a Western context all fat is considered bad. The effect is to place fatness in a dichotomous relationship, between "the West" and "the rest" (Forth 2013, p. 137) and "good" and "bad" fat bodies.

The danger of these "overdrawn oppositions" (Forth 2013, p. 137) and simplistic dichotomies—of what Hardin (2015) (drawing on Mimi Nichter) calls fat-positive and fat-negative talk—is that they speak to an occidentalist discourse in which "the Other" is romanticized and held in temporalities of "tradition." In Othering discourses "far away" and often female bodies are understood through "culture," where kinship, commensality, and reproduction are centrally placed. In Western contexts obesity is understood through discourses that prioritize health and focus on individual bodies and the perceived ills and risks of "modern lives." Such dualist interpretations of traditional/modern and constructs of individual selves and communal Others confine the movement of fat's meanings and materialities within and across cultures, and limit possibilities for thinking of fat and fat bodies outside of a Cartesian trope. Moreover, as McCullough and Hardin note in their book *Reconstructing Obesity*, it seems that fatness can only be valued and thinness avoided in an environment of scarcity—constructing a linear and evolutionary perspective in which fatness decreases in value as development and knowledge increase, thereby placing Euro-American cultural understandings of fatness at the apex of progression.

Ethnographic work, including Amy McLennan's (2013) study of the Pacific island nation of Nauru, Emily Yates-Doerr's work in Guatemala, and Jessica Hardin's (2015) work on fatness and Christianity in Samoa, is beginning to unsettle these rigidly held partitions. In Samoa fatness is associated with mana—sacred power—and fat is seen as evidence of the gods' presence in the life of the individual and the family (Shore 1989). Mana, Hardin writes, is represented "with crude visibility," whether through "height or girth, brightness or generosity; in short, in Polynesia power is expressed though images of abundance"—but this can be interpreted as positive *or* negative according to which type of church people (in this case pastors) are affiliated with (Hardin 2015, p. 184).

Moreover, ethnographic research on disordered eating demonstrates the reasons why people might lose weight (to negate relatedness, manage distress, and fuel desire), and these are not always health-related (see, e.g., Eli 2018; Lavis 2016; Warin 2010). In our field site weight loss was not always motivated by health reasons. Jan, for example, announced one morning that she was going to her son-in-law's wedding: "I have to lose weight. The ex-wife will be there. I know it is petty but I'm determined to lose weight. I've got until April. I'm gonna do it." Ellie laughed, "You only lose weight for weddings," she says. "I know, I know." Jan admits, "but I've got 10 years on that woman and I should shed some weight." Shedding fat here was directly linked to dominant conceptualizations of thinness, and the cultural capital that thinness accrues (especially for women) in Australian society.

In engaging ontological and materialist explorations of bodies, our research fleshes out the agentive nature of fat, extending anthropological analyses that socially construct how fat or other bodily substances are rejected or desired. Our study highlights the multiplicities and inconsistencies of fat—how fat repels and attracts, how its materiality can bring us closer to and create distance from other people and things. Similar to Barad's (2007, 2014) conceptual move from the interactive to the "intra-active," Colls (2007) spatial enquiry into fat plunges into what she terms "embodied topographies" to elicit how fat is "not only impinged upon by outside forces but has its own capacities to act and be active" (2007, p. 358). In Colls' bodily landscape fat can incite positive (and pleasurable) reactions as its multiple layers "gather" in folds and ridges, and fleshy spaces "dance" together in new material formations. Matter, then, in being "implicated in its own materialization" thus prompts "us to consider what matter can do to a body and what it can enable a body to do" (2007, p. 363).

Fat can produce health problems. But the focus on fat solely as health risk undermines its other multiple functions. Fat not only disables, it also enables bodies to do stuff. And fat did many things in the lives of participants. We have traced their agentic accounts to give voice to these productive and positive meanings of fat. We have shown how fat warms bodies, how it nurtures and sustains those living in impoverished circumstances, and cushions them in a world that can be cruel and unkind. Fat also labors to get things in a gendered currency of social and material exchange. We have witnessed the variegation of fat across and within bodies, demonstrating that there are different values accorded to different types of fat that are produced in different classed terrains. It is not only "the body" then but also its constituent parts that are multiple (Mol 2002). Departing from ingrained binary divisions (of the biological and the social, of traditional and modern, and of healthy [thin] bodies and unhealthy [fat] ones), participants' conceptualizations and enactments of fat show us how seemingly conflicting experiences of fat "hang together" (Mol 2002, p. 5), come forward, or remain mute depending on certain contexts.

In campaigning to restrict the consumption of fat, obesity prevention initiatives take aim at fat bodies, or in public health vernaculars those that expand above and beyond a "healthy weight." Designed to excise the substance of fat and reduce the presence of fat people, these programs take for granted a singular, discrete, and passive entity—"fat"—which can be isolated and removed from people's lives as well as bodies. We would argue that attending to this "ontological singularity" (Mol 2002) diminishes the lived, relational experience of fat and its entanglements with other people and things. It omits the existence of multiple fatnesses, discounting how *they* are enacted and how they produce effects (see Bennett 2010, p. 5). It is this wider recognition of the agency of fat—it's multiple ways of being and becoming—in local environments and lives that we suggest needs to be "given weight" in crafting obesity policy and intervention programs.

Note

1. As well as these studies it is important to remember that historians of fat have consistently shown that there have always been alternative readings and positions on fat and fatness in the so-called West (see, e.g., Schwartz 1986; Stearns 2002; Hutson 2017).

References

Abbots, E., & Lavis, A. (2012). *Why we eat, how we eat: Contemporary encounters between foods and bodies.* Farnham: Ashgate.

Aphramor, L. (2005). Is a weight-centred health framework salutogenic? Some thoughts on unhinging certain dietary ideologies. *Social Theory & Health, 3*, 315–340.

Barad, K. (2007). *Meeting the universe halfway: Quantum physics and the entanglement of matter and meaning.* Durham: Duke University Press.

Barad, K. (2014). Posthumanist performativity: Toward an understanding of how matter comes to matter. *Signs, 28*(3), 801–831.

Becker, A. E. (1995). *Body, self, and society: The view from Fiji*. Philadelphia: University of Pennsylvania Press.

Bennett, J. (2007). Edible matter. *New Left Review, 45*, 133–145.

Bennett, J. (2010). *Vibrant matter: A political ecology of things*. Durham: Duke University Press.

Bennett, J. (2011). Powers of the hoard: Artistry and agency in a world of vibrant matter. *Vera List Center for Art and Politics*, [Lecture] *The New School*, New York, 27. Available at http://www.materialworldblog.com/2012/01/jane-bennett-lecture-powers-of-the-hoard-artistry-and-agency-in-a-world-of-vibrant-matter/

Berlant, L. (2010). Risky bigness: On obesity, eating and the ambiguity of health. In J. Metzl & A. Kirkland (Eds.), *Against health: How health became the new morality* (pp. 26–39). New York: New York University Press.

Berlant, L. (2011). *Cruel optimism*. Durham: Duke University Press.

Colls, R. (2007). Materialising bodily matter: Intra-action and the embodiment of 'fat'. *Geoforum, 38*(2), 353–365.

Colls, R. (2012). Big girls having fun': Reflections on a fat accepting space. *Somatechnics, 2*, 18–37.

Dennis, S. (2013). Researching smoking in the new smokefree: Good anthropological reasons for unsettling the public health grip. *Health Sociology Review, 22*(3), 282–290.

Devitt, J. (1991). Traditional preferences in a changed context: Animal fats as valued foods. *Central Australian Rural Practitioners' Association Newsletter, 13*, 16–18.

Edmonds, A. (2010). *Pretty modern: Beauty, sex and plastic surgery in Brazil*. Durham: Duke University Press.

Ehlers, N. (2014). Fat is the future: Bioprospecting, fat stem cells, and emergent breasted materialities. In C. E. Forth & A. Leitch (Eds.), *Fat: Culture and materiality* (pp. 109–122). London: A & C Black.

Eli, K. (2018). Striving for liminality: Eating disorders and social suffering. *Transcultural Psychiatry*. https://doi.org/10.1177/1363461518757799.

Forth, C. (2013). The qualities of fat: Bodies, history, and materiality. *Journal of Material Culture, 18*(2), 135–154.

Forth, C. (2014). Thinking through fat: The materiality of ancient and modern stereotypes. In C. E. Forth & A. Leitch (Eds.), *Fat: culture and materiality* (pp. 53–69). London: A & C Black.

Forth, C., & Leitch, A. (Eds.). (2014). *Fat: Culture and materiality*. London: A & C Black.

Gay, R. (2017). *Hunger: A memoir of (my) body*. New York: Hachette.

Government of South Australia, City of Playford. (2010). *State of the City Report*. http://www.playford.sa.gov.au/webdata/resources/files/State_of_the_City_Report_2010.pdf

Hardin, J. (2015). Christianity, fat talk, and Samoan pastors: Rethinking the fat-positive-fat-stigma framework. *Fat Studies, 4*(2), 178–196.
Hutson, D. (2017). Plump or corpulent? Lean or gaunt? Historical categories of bodily health in nineteenth-century thought. *Social Science History, 41*(2), 283–303.
Kendrick, R. (2013). Metabolism as strategy: Agency, evolution and biological hinterlands. In E. Abbotts & A. Lavis (Eds.), *Why we eat, how we eat: Contemporary encounters between foods and bodies* (pp. 237–254). Farnham: Ashgate.
Lancet, D. E. (2015). Tackling obesity: Is coercion an option? *The Lancet Diabetes and Endocrinology, 3*(4), 227.
Land, N. (2018). Fat knowledges and matters of fat: Towards re-encountering fat(s). *Social Theory & Health, 16*(1), 77–93.
Lavis, A. (2016). A Desire for anorexia: Living through distress. *Medical Anthropology Theory, 3*(1), 68–76.
LeBesco, K. (2004). *Revolting bodies?: The struggle to redefine fat identity.* Amherst: University of Massachusetts Press.
Lupton, D. (2013). *Fat.* London: Routledge.
McDonald, H. (2003). The fats of life. *Australian Aboriginal Studies,* (2), 53–61.
McLennan, A. (2013). *An ethnographic investigation of lifestyle change: Living for the moment, and obesity emergence in Nauru.* Unpublished PhD thesis, University of Oxford.
Mol, A. (2002). *The body multiple: Ontology in medical practice.* London: Duke University Press.
Monaghan, L. (2005). Big handsome men, bears and others: Virtual constructions of 'fat male embodiment'. *Body & Society, 11*(2), 81–111.
Murray, S. (2008). *The 'fat' female body.* Melbourne: Palgrave Macmillan.
Pausé, C. (2017). Candy perfume girl: Colouring in fat bodies. *FKW/Zeitschrift für Geschlechterforschung und visuelle Kultur,* (62). Retrieved from https://www.fkw-journal.de/index.php/fkw/article/view/1403
Pollock, N. (1995). Social fattening patterns in the pacific: The positive side of obesity: A Nauru case study. In I. De Garine & N. J. Pollock (Eds.), *Social aspects of obesity* (pp. 87–110). Luxembourg: Gordon & Breach Publishers.
Popenoe, R. (2004). *Feeding desire: Fatness, beauty and sexuality among a Saharan people.* London: Routledge.
Powdermaker, H. (1960). An anthropological approach to the problem of obesity. *Bulletin of the New York Academy of Medicine, 36*(5), 286–295.
Probyn, E. (2008). IV. Silences behind the mantra: Critiquing feminist fat. *Feminism & Psychology, 18*(3), 401–404.
Redmond, A. (2001). *Rulug Wayirri: Moving kin and country in the northern Kimberley.* Doctoral thesis, University of Sydney.

Reinarman, C. (2005). Addiction as accomplishment: The discursive construction of disease. *Addiction Research & Theory, 13*(4), 307–320.
Renzaho, A. (2004). Fat, rich and beautiful: Changing socio-cultural paradigms associated with obesity risk, nutritional status and refugee children from Sub-Saharan Africa. *Health & Place, 10*(1), 105–113.
Schwartz, H. (1986). *Never satisfied: A cultural history of diets, fantasies and fat.* New York: The Free Press.
Shore, B. (1989). Manu and Tapu. In A. Howard & R. Borofsky (Eds.), *Developments in Polynesian ethnology* (pp. 137–173). Honolulu: University of Hawaii Press.
Sobo, E. (1993). *One blood: The Jamaican body.* New York: SUNY Press.
Sobo, E. (1997). The sweetness of fat. In C. Counihan & P. Van Esterik (Eds.), *Food and culture: A reader* (pp. 256–271). New York: Routledge.
Solovay, S., & Rothblum, E. (2009). Introduction. In E. Rothblum & S. Solovay (Eds.), *The fat studies reader* (pp. 1–10). New York: New York University Press.
Stearns, P. (2002). *Fat history: Bodies and beauty in the modern west.* New York: New York University Press.
Throsby, K. (2013). Guest article: Dr Karen Throsby, on the complicated issue of fat amongst Channel swimmers. LoneSwimmer. https://loneswimmer.com/2013/02/05/guest-article-dr-karen-throsby-on-the-complicated-issue-of-fat-amongst-channel-swimmers/
Throsby, K. (2015). 'You can't be too vain to gain if you want to swim the Channel': Marathon swimming and the construction of heroic fatness. *International Review for the Sociology of Sport, 50*(7), 769–784.
Tove, M. J., Swami, V., Furnham, A., & Mangalparsed, R. (2006). Changing perceptions of attractiveness as observers are exposed to a different culture. *Evolution and Human Behavior, 27*(6), 443–456.
Wann, M. (1998). *Fat! So? Because you don't have to apologize for your size.* Berkeley: Ten Speed Press.
Warin, M. (2010). *Abject relations: Everyday worlds of anorexia.* New Brunswick: Rutgers University Press.
Warin, M. (2015). Material feminism, obesity science and the limits of discursive critique. *Body & Society, 21*(4), 48–76.
Wilson, E. A. (2015). *Gut feminism.* Durham: Duke University Press.
Yates-Doerr, E. (2015). *The weight of obesity: Hunger and global health in postwar Guatemala.* Berkeley: University of California Press.
Zivkovic, T., Warin, M., Moore, V., Ward, P., & Jones, M. (2015). The sweetness of care: Biographies, bodies and place. In E. Abbotts, A. Lavis, & L. Attala (Eds.), *Careful eating: Bodies, food and care* (pp. 109–112). Farnham: Ashgate.
Zivkovic, T., Warin, M., Moore, V., Ward, P., & Jones, M. (2018). Fat as productive: Enactments of fat in an Australian suburb. *Medical Anthropology: Cross Cultural Studies in Health and Illness, 37*(5), 373–386.

CHAPTER 7

Shades of Shame and Pride

On a wintery afternoon in the field Tanya stepped out of a fierce gust of wind to board the train for the 40-minute ride back to the city center. It was early afternoon and she took a seat nearest to two teenage girls, who were huddled together engaged in conversation. Aged around 16 and neither slim nor fat, they both wore skinny-leg jeans and had dip-dyed hair. Quietly animated discussions came to an abrupt end when the train stopped at the Elizabeth station and they gasped in unison, as if confronted by a most repugnant sight. They screwed up their faces with expressions of disgust, their arms flailing about as they laughed and pointed at a corpulent figure who sat with her back to them on the platform. The woman's body was not quite contained in the long bench seat; it was spilling out through the sides. A bulbous mound of flesh was escaping both her tracksuit pants and sweater. A target of ridicule and scorn, this visible, wobbling mound of fat was stared at disdainfully by the two younger women. Stepping from the train, they approached the layers of drooping flab from behind, pretending to vomit as they inched closer and closer to the body, in actions that appeared to go unnoticed by the woman. Then, as if now bored with their performance, they walked away from the woman and casually approached the nearby bus stand.

By acting out their disgust at the sight of a corpulent body, these young women signaled the profound stigma that large bodies in Australian (and most Western countries) endure. The unsuspecting woman on the platform symbolized the horror of corpulence, a body that was culturally "out

M. Warin, T. Zivkovic, *Fatness, Obesity, and Disadvantage in the Australian Suburbs*,
https://doi.org/10.1007/978-3-030-01009-6_7

of bounds" because it overflowed with abundance and flesh (Braziel and LeBesco 2001). Her hyper-visible body failed to physically fit within the public seating and spoke "without necessarily talking because [it was] coded with and as signs … [and was already] intextuated, narrativized, and incarnated with social codes, laws, norms and ideals" (Grosz 1995, p. 35). By not fitting into her clothes and not fitting into the seat, the woman was "publically misfitting" (Brewis et al. 2017), and a target of scorn.

Feminist academic Samantha Murray similarly reflects on this tacit coding in relation to her own experience as a large child, adolescent, and woman. As a critical scholar and fat activist, Murray's writing on fatness comes from a poststructuralist angle and unveils the power relations that are embedded within obesity discourses with their inevitable medicalization and pathologization of fatness. In her book *The Fat, Female Body* (2008), she points to what others describe as a "fraught standpoint" (Throsby and Gimlin 2010, p. 107) between theorizing fat embodiment and recognizing her own experiences of fatness:

> *I was immediately attracted to the fat pride movement, who seemed to take up the idea of intervening in the contract one's fatness has with the world, insisting on being seen in new ways. So, I go out into the world armed with the Fat Manifesto* (Waun 1998), *wearing a sleeveless top, my dimpled arms on display. I feel strong, powerful, swollen with my fat identity, snarling at others who cast withering glances at my bulky frame. And then, I pass a shop window.*
>
> *I shudder as I catch a reflection of myself, my body appearing to me as grotesque and foreign, a bulging, jiggling vehicle of disgust and shame I want nothing to do with. I experience myself/my body in ways that shift and vary and contradict each other.* (Murray 2005, p. 153)

In exploring these public and personal responses to fatness, many scholars draw upon the classic work of sociologist Erving Goffman to discuss the power of "discrediting attributes" (1963/2009). Scholars working on fatness have already explored the role of stigma in relation to obesity (see Brewis et al. 2017; Farrell 2011; Guthman 2009; McCullough 2013; Pausé 2017; Saguy and Ward 2011), and deeply entrenched "fatphobia" (Saguy and Ward 2011). Lupton (2012), for example, drawing directly from Goffman, has articulated the ways in which people are ostracized from society by responses to their "spoiled identities." Spoiled identities are those that draw negative reactions due to their perceived difference to the norm, through conditions such as obesity or mental illness. Societal disapproval leads to social stigma, and "has repercussions for the stigmatized individual in his or her dealings in social life such as exclusion, marginalization, ostracism, social discrimination, and less access to privileged occupations, housing, educational opportunities and so on" (Lupton 2012, p. 26). People who are overweight or obese certainly experience stigma and, like the unknown woman sitting at the train station, "are subjected to abuse, humiliation, and shaming practices, and are portrayed in both medical and popular media as sick, irresponsible, ignorant, and abnormal" (ibid.).

Stigma was a common issue in our field site, but the example of the young girls making fun of a fat woman is only one site of stigma enactment. Stigma works its way in and out of different situations—it can be direct, invisible, and manifest in everyday spaces, societal structures, and institutions. People's responses to stigma will vary according to who they are, their sexuality, age, gender, and ethnicity, and where they are at a particular time in their life course. Goffman's account of stigma is valuable, but here its value is limited, for it is a static and seemingly universal concept that bears down heavily on people. The Obesity Prevention and Lifestyle (OPAL) program acknowledged this heavy burden of stigma that is placed on large people by erasing words and images that point to obesity. But this did not make it disappear. As Derrida (1976) suggests, there is a double gesture in erasure, for when one tries to hide or erase the meaning of a text, it only serves to make visible that which has already been construed. Moreover, as Murray's reflexive piece suggests, stigma is an embodied and relational experience that develops through the interplay of shame and pride.

In this final chapter we explore how shame and pride shifted in bodies according to different contexts, situations, and historical circumstances. Key to this analysis is to identify ways in which shame is shaped by class. Rich et al. (2015) suggest that "one of the most powerful forms of stigmatization and discrimination circulating within contemporary health emerges when the social and cultural tensions of social class intersect with obesity discourse" (Rich et al. 2015, p. 1). Pearl, an Indigenous interviewee we introduced in Chap. 6, reflected on the question of who feels shame when it comes to obesity. She said that middle-class people are more ashamed of fat: "They're the ones who are really bothered by it," whereas "people around here don't spend their lives trying to hide when they get a few bags [of fat]." Other bodily markers of disadvantage, like poor teeth, also had different registers of shame according to context, where sometimes it was unremarkable and at other times could be an indication of a person's unemployability. Bodies in our field site slipped in and out of different daily contexts and were "both objects and subjects" (Mol and Law 2004, p. 43), and hence located in and experiencing differing shades of shame and pride.

One line of argument might suggest that local acts of resistance to obesity interventions are distancing tactics emanating from the stigma that accompanies living in an area that is routinely derided by the media, and the shame of being labeled as a fat person living in a fat community. This resistance is important to acknowledge; however, the community was not homogeneous and fat discrimination is so pervasive that it occurred within the community and was not simply practiced by outsiders.

By attending to the embodiment of shame and pride and drawing on theoretical insights from Probyn (2005) and Tyler (2015), our analysis points to the multiplicity of de-stigmatizing strategies, and their temporal ordering in a range of contexts. This occurred through distancing of Others within the community, comparisons with others worse off or fatter, and a series of compensating strategies designed to "bend the rules" or "milk the system." Many of these resources were of short duration—"making ends meet," "tiding oneself over" with food bank freebies, divvies, or one-off meals. In the final part of the chapter, we look at the pride that came with "breaking the cycle," not described in terms of healthy weight or healthy eating, but rather the resources garnered to enable people to have healthier lives.

Imogen Tyler makes the important point in her paper on class in the UK (2015) that class should not be grounded in the valorization of class identity (such as pride in former working-class identity), but rather class should be understood as "struggles against classification." Lisa McKenzie, in her book *Getting By: Estates, Class and Culture in Austerity Britain* (2015), gives a powerful example. In this work she explores how working-class residents living at St Ann's housing estate in Nottingham develop their own systems of value and comfort (such as purchasing knock-off Gucci sunglasses) which allow them to participate in a consumer society and feel good about themselves. These local economies of value were like adding a "little bit of sugar in [one's] tea" (McKenzie 2015, p. 110). McKenzie describes the complex negotiations that women on the estate grappled with, of how "negative namings, feelings of 'being looked down on', anger and humiliation, are absorbed into the self but can also act as signifying systems to push against" (2015, p. 112). There is a constant battle of outside negativity with insider pride, and reconciling this with "who they are, and how they want to be seen, but also in what they do" (ibid.). These struggles to reconcile pride and shame are what people in our fieldwork spoke to. Shame and pride operated as complex de-stigmatization strategies (Peacock et al. 2014), rallying against being labeled as "obese," "uneducated," "ignorant, unable to care for family," or as "a failure."

Anti-stigma

Several of the stakeholders we interviewed were well aware of the judgments that came hand-in-hand with asking people to change their diets and levels of physical activity. OPAL should be applauded for not reproducing what Charlotte Cooper (2017) refers to as "headless fatties," and the negative emotions of disgust associated with images of fat or fat people (as many previous public health campaigns have done). New Zealand fat activist, Cat Pausé, argues that despite public health awareness of the damaging role of stigma, their campaigns frequently use the power of stigma in anti-obesity campaigns. She details the long history of using graphic imagery to produce fear and disgust in order to scare people into health behavior change. The "Grabbable Gut" marketing from the "Live Lighter" campaign in Western Australia released images of a man grabbing his stomach with both hands, with an adjacent image of yellow fat around internal organs. The accompanying text states that "grabbable gut outside means toxic fat inside" (https://livelighter.com.au/The-Facts/About-Toxic-Fat).

Pausé notes similar campaigns around the world that use confronting and stigmatizing images and text about fat; for example, "the Strong4Life campaign from Children's Healthcare of Atlanta, the 'Pouring on the Pounds' campaign from the New York City Department of Health and Mental Hygiene, and the anti-obesity cheese campaign (Your Thighs on Cheese) from the Physicians Committee for Responsible Medicine" (Pausé 2017, p. 513).

At the outset of OPAL (as mentioned in Chap. 2) there were clear guidelines about the program being non-stigmatizing, and there was a decision not to use the word obesity in the social marketing or brochures that appeared in community spaces.[1] One OPAL manager said: "It can be important to look like you don't have a stigmatizing approach; you don't want to be the 'food Nazi': you want to show that some foods are 'sometimes foods' and that means it is OK to have them sometimes. It's a difficult balance but you don't want people to be made uncomfortable by your presence." All the social marketing themes were consciously branded as "positive, non-stigmatizing messages," and not emphasizing weight or weight loss. There were no images of overweight or obese people in any of this branding.

Despite the public health campaigns that Pausé presents, there are more positive examples of how the symbolic burden (Farrugia 2011) of the word obesity is navigated in international obesity campaigns (Warin and Gunson 2013). Like OPAL, the UK's Change4Life program (2009–2011) invested millions of pounds to address rising obesity rates (Evans et al. 2011; Piggin and Lee 2011). This was a huge public health campaign, which the UK's Department of Health described as delivering on a "scale never previously witnessed" (p. 6). Ironically, as Piggin and Lee (2011) point out, the campaign did not mention obesity, the very problem it was trying to address.

Bombak et al. (2016) refer to this deliberate non-stigmatizing approach as the "mainstream approach ... propagated by health agencies, groups and some scholarly literature" (2016, pp. 94–95). In this approach obesity should be addressed and "policy, programming and research must focus on the eradication of excess fat from populations, but that individuals with obesity should not be discriminated against for body types beyond their control" (2016, p. 95). Weight reduction was one measurable goal for the program, but public brochures and marketing did not mention obesity (preferring less-stigmatizing terms like "healthy weight"). The omission of the word obesity is not an intentionally deceptive omission, but speaks to a desire to not further marginalize people. This has led to a rather tricky positioning whereby obesity was both remarkably present *and* absent: it was managed carefully to be hidden in conversations, social marketing, and in the daily routines of OPAL workers.

The second approach to stigma that Bombak et al. (2016) identify is in line with critical scholars who argue that obesity stigma is "fully and completely embedded in the notion that 'excess' fat is unhealthy, and the only way to end fat-based discrimination is to stop presenting fatness as always-already insalubrious" (Bombak et al. 2016, p. 95). This is the intellectual space that Samantha Murray inhabits, the collective knowingness about all fat bodies—what Murray calls a "constant silent presumption" (2005, p. 154). This assumed knowingness about fat bodies is so diffuse that any obesity intervention program, by its very nature, cannot seek to overcome the influence of fat prejudice.

This means that it is impossible to step outside of the ways in which fat bodies are already deeply imbued with value. When we perceive a body as fat, we constitute it in accordance with the bodily knowledges that provide a backdrop for our perception (Murray 2007, p. 362). How we perceive and understand each other is thus hidden and tacit, as Murray (2007) explains:

> *[These tacit knowledges are] inferred without being directly expressed; they are habitual and embodied without any conscious decisions made about deploying them at any given moment. In other words, we respond to each other in a visceral level: we know their bodies implicitly, and what they mean to us. We see a "fat" woman, and we know her to be lazy, greedy, of inferior intelligence.* (Murray 2007, p. 363)

Despite the absence of the word obesity in the OPAL marketing for the community, there was no hiding the fact that community members knew that OPAL was about obesity—"It's about 'don't be a couch potato'; to help people eat healthy ... to help the whole of Playford know what fruit is." The message OPAL pronounced spoke to a lack of awareness, education, and knowledge about healthy eating and activity, emphasizing the need to "meet guidelines," to "improve," to "make better choices," to make "good choices," and to "reduce" and "replace" current food items and activities. The message was clear that people needed to change "the 'wrong' behaviors." While obesity wasn't mentioned, the messages all pointed to a *lack*—which is precisely what obese people are accused of (lack of control, lack of knowledge, lack of discipline). One stakeholder admitted that "[w]hen people look at those [OPAL] brochures about obesity, they think 'shit, that's me' and feel bad. We are just disempowering them further. Obesity is a complex problem that requires complex solutions and nobody knows how to tackle it. The obvious solution of talking to people hasn't bloody occurred to anyone." OPAL's moralizing messages only highlighted class disparities: between community members, with their priorities for feeding families "from payday to payday" on a limited budget, and the relatively privileged government workers who sought to reshape their pantries and their bodies.

* * *

There is a long history of the working classes being subject to targets of self-improvement by the middle to upper classes. Tyler (2015) notes that Angela McRobbie has for quite some time detailed the "public humiliation of people for their failure to adhere to middle-class standards in speech or appearance [that] has become acceptable and normalized in ways that would have been considered offensive, discriminatory or prejudicial" in the postwar welfarist period (McRobbie 2005, p. 100, cited in Tyler 2015, p. 503). Despite the political and popular retreat from class (and silencing of the topic via accusations of "class welfare"), social scientists have systematically been documenting and commenting on the "deserving poor and the rest, who [are] morally condemned for their ecklessness and immorality" (Bourdieu 2000, p. 79).

People in our field site dealt with what you might call intersectional stigmatization (c.f. Puhl and Heuer 2010, p. 1021)—of low socioeconomic status, of higher incidence of being overweight and obese, of higher than average crime rates, of high unemployment, and even of denigration concerning family composition (higher than average numbers of single-parent households). Class is particularly relevant here, as Bombak et al. (2016) note: "Obesity stigma is a stand in or a re-articulation of other forms of oppressions, such as class" (p. 95). Even when middle to upper classes are asked about the "the problem of obesity" in Australia, the immediate recourse is to a narrative of the "Other," "those people" living in circumstances of disadvantage (Farrell et al. 2016; Carey et al. 2017).

Running alongside this stigmatization, and almost in the same breath, was a focus on community pride in the face of adversity. Pride and community solidarity was a common discourse we heard in the field (articulated in different ways by community members and local government workers), and exemplified by social historian Peel's summation:

> *People living in Elizabeth's poorest neighborhoods already have a strong sense of identity and solidarity which might in fact make them a community. They have all the dense networks of self-help and sharing of resources, a sense of mutual needs and problems, highly localized solidarities and local activisms centered on schools, neighborhood houses and other small-scale institutions. What they haven't got is money, jobs, or much sense of a future.* (Peel 1995, p. 235)

Many of these forms of solidarity were evident in the range of community and welfare services, from cheap, hot meals provided by various organizations, free financial advice, food banks, alcohol and mental health services, domestic violence services, support for the homeless, and free legal advice. People from the North sense an allegiance through their shared location and often their shared predicaments. If you are from the North you might be expected by some locals to speak a certain way (to say "haff," not "have") and identify as "a Norfie." If you shop at the food bank, this generates relationships and acknowledgment of shared day-to-day struggles. In our fieldwork we saw strangers on a train strike up a casual friendship based on their self-identification of "not having much," when one man said to another passenger whom he had just met: "Like you and me my friend, like you and me."

Other less formal types of solidarity were also evident, and these were individual acts of "everyday resistance" (Scott 1985/2008) against class positionings. People talked about "milking, gaming, and cheating the system," as ways to make a buck and hold (if only momentarily) a bit of power. This did not take the form of collective or public protests, but sly, sometimes criminal, acts, such as stealing the copper piping from the public toilets in the main shopping center (copper can be sold for a good price at local sheet metal works) or stealing a cheesecake from a shop. There was much discussion about "sussing out the welfare system," because "people round here know how to rort the system … they abuse the system. They know how it works, they use it to the max." All of these small acts of resistance demonstrated ways to extract a little power amid the daily grind of struggle.

In our research it was only the OPAL staff who talked about stigma. Stigma was not a word that participants used; rather, they would sometimes talk about how others saw them and the ways in which they were "put down" by others. Rather than stigma, their discourse revealed a constant interplay of shame and pride. Participants talked about "getting by," "living poor," and "making ends meet," and the short-term strategies that they used to stretch budgets and food to make things last.[2] These "stretching and bending" activities (along with "milking the system") were a source of pride, and were ways to feel good in the struggle against adversity and precarity. A number of participants spoke to imagined lives beyond "making ends meet," and how they could break the cycle of disadvantage through structural changes in employment and new education opportunities. All of these de-stigmatization strategies (whether short term or more sustained in and across family lives) generated pride against the shame of being labeled as fat and poor (c.f. Lister 2004).

Shame, Pride, and De-stigmatizing Strategies

In her book *Blush*, Probyn (2005) examines the complex workings of shame, arguing that "something about shame is terribly important. By denying or denigrating it or trying to eradicate it (as in countless self-help books written to counter various strains of shame), we impoverish ourselves and our attempts to understand human life" (2005, p. 3). Shame is a difficult emotion to investigate, and one reviewer of Probyn's work had trouble with the many personal anecdotes that she used to locate and prize shame out of her body (Holmes 2006). But this is where shame resides: it lurks in bodies, in emotions. Importantly, for our fieldwork, Probyn brings to the fore the ways in which shame is not simply a negative state, but a feeling, emotion, and affect which plays on a "fine line or border between moving forward into more interest or falling back into humiliation" (Probyn 2005, p. xii).

Shame and pride are intimately entangled and cannot be easily separated. Fat pride is but one example of a long line of historical "pushing back" against the shame of spoiled identities, also to be seen in the contemporary politics of being gay (gay pride) and racism (black pride). In this context, pride works to eradicate shame and comes to the fore as a positive emotion to embody. Candy, for example, from Chap. 6, is proud of "her girls": her fleshy breasts that "get her things." Probyn argues, however, that shame cannot be completely erased; it sticks to bodies and becomes deeply engrained.

Like the word stigma, shame was not a term that we heard in the field. Shame might be unspoken but is embodied and experienced in and through the body. We observed how some people came into the food banks, sometimes speaking to each other in whispers and avoiding eye contact, and at other times fidgeting with coins in their pockets and hanging back, hesitant to come forward and speak to volunteers. Others were very much at home in the food bank, laughing and joking with volunteers, seeking advice about bureaucratic forms to be filled in, or how to pay bills. Sometimes volunteers commented on a person's appearance: a thin body draped in ill-fitting clothes, or tight garments stretched to the seams trying to hold flesh in. Hunger and malnutrition (embodied as a dual burden of underweight or overweight/obesity) were both markers of shame, pride, and hard times.

Children were singled out as particular markers of shame: their unruly behaviors, the lack of shoes, or unkempt bodies signaling that mothers (most often characterized as "single mothers") were unable to afford clothes or food. One volunteer in the food bank described a family that used to come into the shop on a regular basis:

> *There was this mother who would come in here with her two kids. They were young like 2, 3 or 4 years old. They were always dirty and I mean real dirty and their hair was always a total mess, just like birds' nests. They looked like they had not bathed in weeks and their clothes were always tattered and cheap and nasty and ill-fitting, as though straight from the second-hand shop. The girl didn't even have underwear on. They were thin too, real thin. The mother would speak to them horribly. Whenever they came in I wanted to take them home. I wanted to give them a bath and wash their hair and give them fresh, new, clean clothes and a good nutritious home-cooked meal and a lovely warm bed. Oh, how I wanted to do that for them! Every time they came in, Jan would just look at me and say "Don't say a thing."*

Like obesity, these types of material deprivations are publicly written on bodies, and read by many as signs of bad mothering. In her discussion of poverty and class in the USA, Adair (2002) details the many inscriptions or signals that become embodied in the spiraling cycles of poverty. She describes her own struggles at finding the money to pay the bills, selling her blood at two or three different clinics each month in order to put shoes on her daughter's feet. She became so anemic that the blood banks refused to buy it from her. A neighbor of hers was left with no other option but to return to the man who was beating her, as she was denied welfare benefits and could not "adequately feed, clothe and house her children" (Adair 2002). Poverty in our field site is inscribed in local biologies (Lock 1993) and in "the imperfect bodies of the poor" (Peel 2004): in crooked backs, missing teeth, and prematurely aged, frail, or obese bodies. Ill-fitting shoes and hand-me-down clothes, dull skin, constant sickness, and crooked, ill-serviced teeth are read, in Foucauldian terms, as texts "juxtaposed against a logic of normative subjectivity as the embodiment of dependency, disorder, disarray and Otherness" (Adair 2002, pp. 461–462).

Bodily Injuries of Class

In the field we became particularly aware of teeth, or rather the absence of them among many of the customers in the food bank. Teeth were sometimes graying, worn down to stubs, or missing altogether. A grandmother in her early 50s recalled a story of how one Christmas all four of her bottom teeth fell out. "They just snapped" she recounted. "There was no pain and I guess I should be happy about that but I was pretty disappointed, I mean Christmas day and I lost all my bloody teeth!" Now she has dentures and, like other participants in the field, there are many foods that she couldn't eat because of her lack of teeth and dentures, like pork crackling, or anything hard, like apples. "I couldn't bite into an apple, for instance, because my dentures would just fall out."

We wondered how people felt about having missing teeth and what they thought about others whose teeth were missing. These thoughts were particularly salient when an exceptionally thin woman about 40 years old came in to the food bank one afternoon with a Salvos voucher and tried to build up her shopping to be exactly $30. "Why don't you take the apples?" says Jan. "We'll give you all those for a dollar." There seemed to be around 3 kg of apples in the prepackaged bag. The woman looked to her teenage daughter, who herself had a young daughter in a stroller. "Well *I* can't eat them but you might, or little missy," she said, pointing to her granddaughter. As the woman talked, we noticed she only had a handful of graying teeth in her mouth.

At a local shopping center where OPAL was running a community session on the best ideas for improving healthy eating, a very large man in his 60s, with an English accent and graying teeth, suggested: "The best idea you could have here to help people eat better is a good dental service. Take me, I cannot bite into an apple. It is much easier to pick up and eat an apple than it is to make a sandwich, but I just can't do it." When teeth start to decay they are painful, and eating becomes difficult. When teeth fall out, the mouth can collapse inward, forcing a person to eat only soft foods, which can lead to poor nutrition.

The man then recounted how costly fixing teeth is. "It would cost $70 that I do not have, that's how much it cost to fix my dentures when I damage them. I know because I've done it four times. We've got no health cover so dental is expensive." His overweight wife chipped in: "I had my bottom dentures done four years ago. I'll need to get the top ones done too." She was missing her front teeth. "But we can't afford the dental. It was OK when we were working because we had private health but he was laid off when he was 40 and we've had no health cover since." Participants often spoke about wishing to have their teeth fixed, and the social status that came with having better teeth. While the cost might be prohibitive for themselves, some would scrimp and save to have a child fitted with braces in order to avoid the shame of crooked teeth. "It cost me a fortune but she has beautiful teeth," said one mother, "It took me years to pay for them."

Being toothless or having missing teeth, maybe more than obesity, was a marker of social disadvantage, of "not looking after yourself." It was a bodily characteristic that sat uncomfortably with potential employers. Even in the food bank, volunteers with no teeth or graying teeth who called in looking for work were seen as not employable or not presentable. Teeth are not only makers of oral hygiene, but markers of class and poverty. Like fat bodies, rotting or missing teeth are the "not so hidden injuries of class" (Adair 2002; Sennett and Cobb 1972), exemplified in the public spectacle of television shows like *Britain's Worst Teeth*, where people from lower socioeconomic areas are shamed for the poor state of their teeth. Adair argues that missing teeth are signs of chaos and indecency: "When my already bad teeth started to rot and I was out of my head with pain, my choices as an adult welfare recipient were either to let my teeth fall out or to have them pulled out. In either case the culture would then read me as a toothless illiterate" (2002, p. 458).

The shame attached to loss of teeth is directly related to health inequities that are deeply embedded in everyday lives. High cost of dental services, poor nutrition, high drug use, and priorities other than oral hygiene mean that many people in this community struggle to attain a level of health that others might reach easily. Citing Sayer (2005) Peacock et al. (2014) argue that there is an expectation that people living in disadvantage can "compete on the same terms as other classes. But without the same resources and advantages they are more likely to fail, to be seen to have failed, and experience themselves as failing—a process [Sayer refers to] as 'structural humiliation'" (Sayer 2005, p. 161, cited in Peacock et al. 2014, p. 392). This embodiment of the shame of structural humiliation requires protections to be drawn, to prevent the insidious nature of shame embedding itself further into bodies, and for resistances to be mounted. We now turn to the ways in which shame was negotiated, distanced, and performed in the field.

Othering and Comparisons

In Chap. 3 we described the social hierarchies within the community. These layers were used as forms of Othering, for labeling certain sections of the community as the "lowest of the low" was a way to distance stigma and shame from oneself. This Othering was most apparent with certain groups, notably mothers who were perceived to be not looking after their children, "druggies," "really fat" people, who were described as lazy and looking for free handouts, and outright racism directed toward immigrants. Angela, a volunteer in the food bank, commented: "Some people around here have no ambition, no drive." She explained how, even though she is on benefits now, she "worked [her] whole life," comparing herself to others who "are lazy and unmotivated." Her husband is on a disability pension and Angela receives $200 per week: "It's quite a struggle but we make ends meet." Again, she compared herself to a very overweight woman she knows who is on a government benefit and who eats three chocolate bars for breakfast and buys takeaway for lunch. "She complains she's got no money and then she goes looking for handouts, the vouchers from Salvos." This story serves to position Angela as similar to this woman (as they are both on the unemployment benefit known as Newstart), but not like her, as she wastes her money and then seeks more handouts. In this context Angela projects herself as a good citizen because she has a history of working and paying tax, and now she spends her benefits wisely, while also contributing to society by working 15 hours a week. "I don't know what the answer is for those people who spend their money on rubbish food. I guess the government should give them less or they should have to work more for it."

Often, after a family had been in the food bank, a story was recounted to explain the background details of their hardship or woes. After one quite large woman had come in on her mobility scooter with her two grandchildren (one of whom was overweight) to buy biscuits, coffee, and milk, Katie turned and said to us:

> *That's the sort of family I mean—they go to all the OPAL events but the message doesn't get through. Those kids are getting bigger and bigger and the mother—you should see their mother, she is really obese. Their mother is the one who came to the first Kids in the Kitchen class here a few weeks back. The one who was eating the hamburgers and wanted the kids to get more for her. That family are just using OPAL for the free handouts. They have the OPAL-installed veggie patch and they come along for free food. I think for them OPAL is just a free lunch and not much else. I think the community, most of them, well they just think of OPAL as a free hand-out. They can get some free food, like kebabs and often fruit, which many of them don't even like, but that's what OPAL is to most of the people here because the OPAL staff go to all the community events and supply food. They might supply other things too: water containers and things like that, frisbees and even for some families veggie gardens in their backyards. So there are some people who just make the most out of it. They go to the OPAL events for a kebab and the freebies but that doesn't mean they make*

any change to their lifestyles. I've been in this business for a long time and I can tell you there is little change. It is very difficult to make any change. I'm not even sure that you can make any change to someone else's behavior: it's very difficult.

Some condemnations heard from community members were extremely harsh, such as suggesting that mothers seen with dirty, unkempt, and too thin children "should be sterilized." On one occasion they described a group of migrant women in the food bank as "like vultures," instantly dehumanizing them with that comparison. Tanya recalls one morning at the food bank when some women of middle-Eastern appearance came in wearing hijabs. On entering the shop they moved straight to the vegetables, which were being sold for $1 a bag. Ellie, the volunteer, watched them and her face wore a sour look as they rummaged through the crates on the floor and on the table near the front counter. "Those women," Ellie said under her breath, "[t]hey want to get as much as possible and pay as little as possible. They just come in for the cheap stuff," she says. Jan agrees. "Oh Tanya, you should see them. Sometimes there are more of them and they are so rude—they try and get a cheaper price by bringing in their own bigger bags. They are like vultures. It is really quite disgusting." The women combine mushrooms, potatoes, and chilies into one of the shop's plastic bags before bringing it to the counter. There is none of the general chitchat between them and the other staff in the shop that is often heard to occur with even the newest of Anglo-looking customers.

This Othering within the community was also something that Shildrick and colleagues noted in their study of poverty across working lives in northeast England. "Even those in the most disadvantaged of circumstances will tend to distance themselves from others who are argued to be 'worse off'" (2010, pp. 37–38). This Othering is a strategy to distance oneself from the broader stigmatizing effects of shame that are directed to those living in disadvantaged situations, making space between us and those like us but not like us. In a community where everyday shame is wrapped up in representations of place, Othering is a struggle to distance oneself from and protect against shame.

This Othering also occurred in relation to body size, with comparisons made between those who were fat and those who were "*really* fat." One day, while buttering bread for lunch in the food bank, Jan recalled: "I don't remember where I was but the other day I was sitting down somewhere—at some meeting I guess—and there was the biggest woman there, and I was transfixed, I couldn't help but look at her overhang. I know it's not nice but I'm honest, it just caught my attention. It was massive. I know I'm fat but I am just nothing compared to this woman. While I was looking at her hips, I started to wonder how big I was, you know, in comparison, and so I kept on feeling my arse to see how big it was as I was looking at hers"; she said this, as she repeated the motion with a hand under each bum cheek, feeling for the distance between where her flesh ended and where the chair began. June laughed: "You don't have to travel far to see some really fat people out here. I saw a man yesterday at the shops and he was so fat I was surprised he could even move." Peta, Jan, and June all nodded together as if perpetually amazed by the size of some bodies. Paul was silent throughout the conversation. He and Tanya were the only non-overweight people sitting at the table: Jan, Peta, and June would all have body mass indexes (BMIs) in the obese category. This everyday conversation of comparison was a way of checking a register or sliding scale of fatness.

"What's on My Divvies?"

In tandem with Othering and comparisons was the practice of bending and stretching, giving people that little bit of extra room to make ends meet. This is something that the workers in the food bank often did, and some practices were done in secret (such as giving away free foods, or delivering foods to people who could not get to the shops), as they knew that would be disapproved of by local council. These sorts of practices were creative, compassionate, and, ultimately, ways to de-stigmatize the shame of having no money to feed yourself or your family.

The food bank had a creative scheme to help people who had little or no money to make ends meet: something to "take the edge off" or provide a single meal, staving off hunger for another day. Our field notes illustrate a typical daily encounter.

> *Tuesday 26 February 2013. Food Bank (field notes)*
>
> *A woman with gray hair comes in looking stoned and disheveled. She stands in front of the coffee for what seems to be a long period then picks up a small bag of the Nescafe. Slowly, languidly, she walks up to the counter, drops it next to the register and speaks with a rough, cracked, and croaky voice: "I wanna pay with my divvies." Unable to remember her number we check her on the system by the first few letters of her surname. She has around $4 in divvies and uses that to pay for her coffee.*

Divvies are the local name given to dividends, the small cents that members can accrue when they shop at either of the two food banks. To become a member you need to pay $10 up front, but as this is a lot of money for many customers, it can be paid for with your divvies as you earn them. Members receive 5% dividends when they purchase items from the food bank, and these can be redeemed at any time. During fieldwork many customers came in to the food banks and asked: "What's on my divvies?" Each member had an assigned number. Regular staff knew shoppers' divvie numbers by heart, and other volunteers would look them up on the computer. Shoppers might use just their divvies, or add it to the small change in their pockets, buying essential items like sanitary products, a small bag of washing powder, or biscuits. This is how one food bank manager described it to us:

> *People come in and ask us what they have, what's their dividend, their share and often people are running short on money, like they don't have the last few cents or they mightn't even have anything and they've got $2 in dividends or more, or whatever amount, and they can use that to buy something, just to tide them over for that moment. I think that's a huge benefit here. That's the philosophy of the Food [bank], that everyone is a member. You all buy in and you're in it together. I advise people not to pay up front in case they decide for whatever reason not to shop here anymore: they might move house for instance—people move around a lot—or for whatever reason and it would be best for that money to stay in their own pockets. So I tell them to let the dividends pay for the membership. A lot more people used to come here but since the redevelopment many of those people no longer come. Much of the public housing has been knocked down. Before, there would be a lot of people who came here without a car—they'd walk here with their kids—but now if those families have been moved out to Salisbury or Gawler they're not going to come here: they're not going to come here by bus, or walk from there.*

Divvies are stopgaps to help people when they literally have just a few cents left till the next payday. Like McDonald's "loose change menu," relished by some participants for cheap ($2) hamburgers, divvies exemplify the struggles that many households constantly face in efforts to feed themselves and their families.

Studies of people who use food banks repeatedly show that they are associated with stigma and shame (Douglas et al. 2015; Garthwaite et al. 2015; Garthwaite 2016). Hannah Lambie-Mumford's work on Britain's fast-growing food bank industry reports that "[f]eelings of embarrassment and stigma, the religious materiality of the spaces in which this food is often provided, and discourses of the 'needy' and the 'hungry' all serve to alienate and socially exclude those in need of assistance with food" (2018, p. 13). Despite food banks becoming normalized in many liberal welfare economies, Garthwaite (2016) and Caplan (2016) claim that people using food banks see themselves as "failures ... and often claim to be ashamed that they cannot provide for their families" (Caplan, cited in Garthwaite 2016, p. 136). At times we were horrified at the state of some food delivered to the food bank—black bananas and organic produce so limp that farm animals might even turn their noses up at it. Shoppers might have been too ashamed to say anything, but the volunteers did comment on the poor quality of the food. Staff often worked out of hours and against the clock trying to salvage rotting food, wrapping leafy green vegetables in cling wrap, making cakes from old bananas, and freezing bakery goods that were beginning to go off. But some food was not salvageable and required disposing. As one manager exclaimed, "[w]e cannot give this food to the poor. Just because they are poor does not mean they should be given moldy food. That's insulting!"

Our work with children on a partner project in the same area (Gunson et al. 2016, 2017) highlighted how food charity was intimately linked to how they located themselves in the world. At a before and after school service in the area we witnessed how the children were acutely aware of the stigma associated with food that came from relief agencies. Receiving food from trucks emblazoned with hunger relief agency signs came with a knowingness that the provision of this food was special, and that by consuming it the children were being marked out as special in some way too. Children would comment on this special status of their food. One young boy said matter-of-factly: "They give us out-of-date food here." On another occasion, when children were given Qantas airline cartons of drinking water that were past their best before date, a girl asked why they were given water "in these weird things" (Gunson et al. 2017). Such subtleties in the processes of marginalization in contexts of socioeconomic deprivation are very important in understanding how experiences of food (including the flavors and textures of out-of-date foods) affect the development of these children's sense of identity and status in the world.

Like Garthwaite, we argue that people use food banks because they do not have choice in what or how they eat. "Necessity," Garthwaite suggests, "not the luxury of choice, means that people are forced to eat food that is cheap, readily available and will not go to waste" (2016, p. 134).

Such "tastes of necessity" meant that people struggled to get by, but alongside and intermingled with this struggle was a pride in resisting shame, demonstrated through what Peacock et al. (2014) refer to as "de-stigmatization strategies."

Tastes of Necessity

A major underpinning tenet of public health prevention efforts is the taken-for-granted capacity of people to look to the future and thus be motivated to mitigate future risks associated with obesity. If presented with health risks, like diabetes or cardiovascular disease, preemptive action can be taken to defuse this anticipated time bomb. OPAL seeks to manage a potentially threatening obesogenic environment by creating conditions in which community members can internalize and act in accordance with shared moral norms about the future benefits of healthy lifestyles (Carter et al. 2011, pp. 57–58).

This politics of temporality (Warin et al. 2015), however, is experienced differently according to social class. Backett-Milburn et al. (2010) show in their study of middle-class teenagers' eating habits in Scotland that middle-class families have future-oriented "hierarchies of luxury and choice," in which controlling and molding teenagers' food practices and tastes was assigned high priority. In comparison, we found that our participants' perceptions of the future were constrained by short horizons, were often fatalistic and unimaginable, with time experienced in the here and now, and as day-to-day. Narrowed vistas of future possibilities led to improvisational practices that clearly circumscribed participants' abilities to respond to OPAL messages. While these "biographies of disadvantage" (Graham et al. 2006) were discordant with the synoptic time of public health futures, it was not that people didn't have hopes or aspirations for the future but rather that they were shaped by the reality of the present. This meant that their opportunities to do and create were limited and situational: they only grasped what was in reach.

One participant, Yvette, illustrated how she extended the present through meticulous attention to budgeting and food management in her home. On our first visit to her house, we were sharply reminded about the arrival of unknown visitors, often presumed to be from welfare or government departments. Walking up to the old South Australian Housing Trust (SAHT) maisonette a woman calls out from the side of the house. She and a man are closing the gates to the backyard. "Tanya is that you? Don't move love. I've got three ex-security dogs and they'll eat you. They're not chained up. Stay there." We froze, afraid to move. We heard the dogs beating against the fence and the sound of metal chains being wound around the gates and secured with padlocks. A security camera faced the front door; it was dated and looked broken. When the front door opened Yvette emerged. A woman in her forties, she was short and her long hair was tied up in a messy ponytail. She had a walking stick and moved unsteadily with a limp, welcoming us in: "Let's sit. It has been one of those crazy days."

Once inside and having been introduced to the three cats, a younger man started to make noises in another room like he was throwing things around. It sounded as if he was throwing furniture around. "What's up Rodney?" Yvette called out as we sat down in the lounge. He yelled back: "Who the hell is this that we've got here now? Who the bloody hell is this?" Yvette explains that they'd had a lawyer visiting earlier on to help with a custody case for her brother's daughter. Her brother is in jail and has asked Yvette to look after his 7-year-old, as her mother "is a real nut-case" and "always tells her she is fat and gives her very little to eat." Yvette is trying to get full custody of the child as she believes the mother and father are unfit parents. This is the picture she paints of the child:

> *When she came here she was so dirty, she had nothing, just the clothes on her back. Really she was just filthy. She did not know words like play or toys. We had to teach her these things. She could not understand why we put food on the table for her three times a day or why we wanted her to have a bath daily. All of these things were new to her.*

Yvette sees herself as a survivor, with the ability to care for others. Self-described as the Jamie Oliver of Playford, she lives on an extremely limited budget. She proudly opened her kitchen cupboards, encouraging us to document this pride. "Take a photo—go on!" she said, revealing every inch of shelf space crammed with a wide range of foods, including long-life products, cans of vegetables, and packet mixes. On each cupboard door was a pantry stock list, an inventory of food items kept updated from month to month. Yvette separated from her husband 15 years ago and raised two children on just $69 a fortnight, so she had to learn to "live poor." In this learning she imagined that she was living in the time of the Great Depression, and that any money or food she had could be her last. She said: "You've got to think that you've got nothing. … It's called survival instinct" (Warin et al. 2015) (Fig. 7.1).

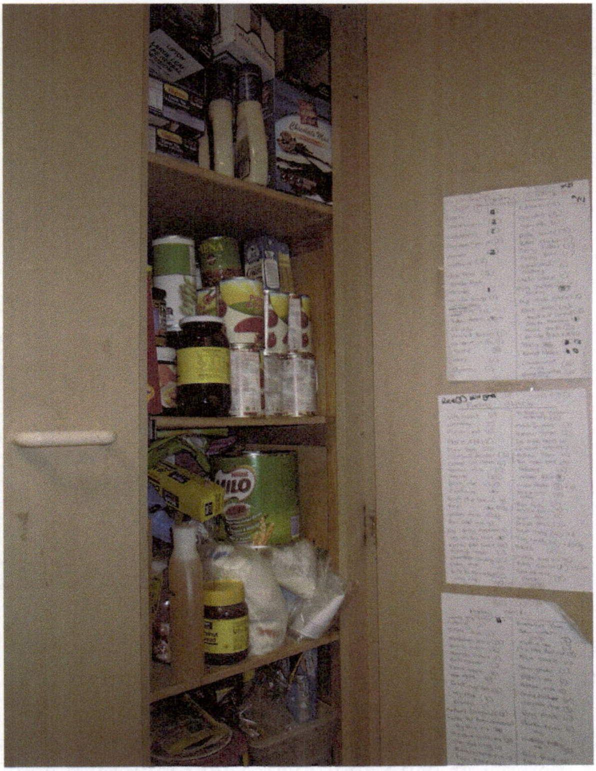

Fig. 7.1 Yvette's well-stocked pantry/cupboard. (Photo from Authors)

Living poor involved eating meat otherwise sold as dog food at the butcher's, and cooking it for as long as possible to make it palatable. Along with such cheap cuts of meat, Yvette might make mashed potato for Rodney's lunch, proudly stating that she could make a meal for 20 cents. She always asked shop staff for packaged and canned foods that had passed their best before dates. In her kitchen she cooked from small appliances, including a gas camping stove on top of her electric cooker as it was a cheaper way to cook. Everyday energy costs are notoriously high in South Australia, and by cooking meals that did not use a lot of gas, instead relying on a quick-cooking pressure cooker, Yvette worked out that she could save A$180 per quarter (Fig. 7.2).

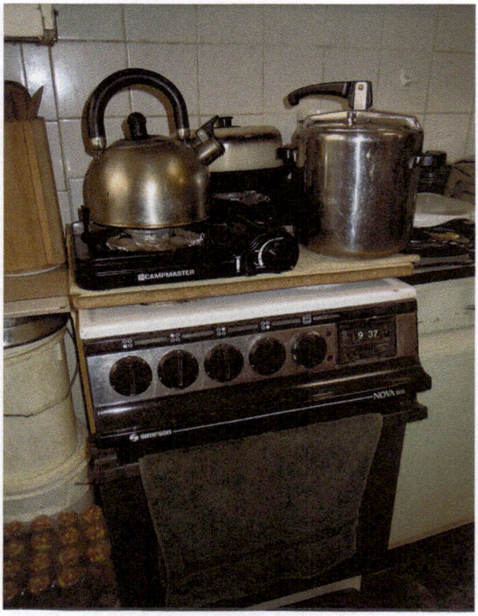

Fig. 7.2 Yvette's camping stove on her kitchen cooker. (Photo from Authors)

These approaches to food, shopping, and cooking were not about healthy eating or tastes of freedom. These were tastes of necessity. Yvette explained that "[i]t was not a choice—it was, 'Okay. I've got to survive. I've got two kids.' ... You've got to concentrate on survival." Yvette reached for material at hand and opened up temporal potentialities that were available in her world.

Yvette was proud of her capacity to survive. People would say to her: "How do you manage to get this, and how do you manage to do that? How do you manage to get bargains? How do you manage to have food in the house? How do you manage to survive ... I can't even survive the fortnight with this, you know? I can't do that." Yvette said she knew a lot of people who rely on short-term measures. She continued: "They get paid on a Thursday but by the Friday they're broke. They walk in on the Monday and they get food assistance. Or they turn around and every three months they rely on the food assistance. They put it as part of their budget. It's just wrong."

Yvette was keen to be involved in local education, providing "basic tips for a survival guide," reminiscent of UK activist Jack Monroe's work on poverty and hunger.[3] Excited about her local knowledge, advice tumbled with ease from her mouth:

> *You can make something out of nothing, you know? If you have potatoes, eggs and pasta in the house, you can turn around and make a poor man's meal with pasta. You cut up the pasta, you turn around, the pasta you boil, you cut up the potatoes, you fry them with a little bit of butter or oil, right, then with that you make a stock, right? Salt and pepper. Then you turn around, you chuck your pasta in, your pasta swells, you chuck your eggs in, that's it. You've got yourself a broth. Just basic, simple things like that. If you've got ham or bacon and a kilo of peas, you mix the two together until the peas turn green or the water turns green and then you chuck your pasta in. If you've got some cheese, a bit of parmesan, that's it. You've got some basic, you know, basic food the Italians used to eat, a poor man's pasta. Chick peas. You boil the chick peas with onions, a bit of garlic, chuck the pasta in, a bit of cheese and you've got another meal. That's next to nothing. Just—I did a lot of homework on the Internet, ring up the rellies, get things down.*

Other participants also proudly shared their strategies for surviving on a limited income. Twenty-five-year-old Fred routinely cooked for other young unemployed men he shared a house with, earning him the title of house mum. Feeding a family on a budget was a role with which Fred was intimately familiar and it was shaped by the cycles of paydays, oscillating between having nothing in terms of meals to overcompensating by providing extra food to his household. As a young child Fred learned to "make little things go a long way" in cooking for a family of eight people with inadequate resources when his parents were on heroin and unable to cook. Fred asserted that it is important to buy extra and on paydays he will stock up on pasta, noodles, meat, and vegetables, the staple and substantial foods used in his regular "cook-ups." Overcooking/overeating is a practical strategy used to offset scarcity by providing whatever one can in the present, knowing that to nurture others and protect them from hunger you overfeed them now (Warin et al. 2015, p. 314).

Yvette and Fred (and other families) demonstrate that many people on low incomes take a highly responsible attitude toward budgeting and purchasing food. This seems to be at odds with the constant push to educate people in circumstances of disadvantage about budgeting for food purchases. Green et al. (2009) similarly found, in their work on families and food in the UK, that budgetary constraints take precedence over everyday choices and purchases, so mothers tended not to experiment with foods that their children might not eat as it meant food was wasted. For families in our research, it was much easier and more cost-saving to choose foods that they knew kids would eat and that are more filling, like burgers and chips (Dobson et al. 1994; Dowler 1997). Rikkie, an overweight mother of two in her early 30s, told us that the food she prepared was "plain Jane" so as to appeal to her children's tastes. With family meals regularly consisting of chicken nuggets, noodles, or hot-dogs, she could ensure her children were fed and that she did not waste money.

Children in our study often remarked that they only eat breakfast cereal covered in sugar, and many said they did not like the taste of the bland cereal promoted by OPAL. Two children aged five and six were quick to express their lack of interest in healthy breakfast options, saying they "couldn't eat it like that. You need sugar." One mother of five reechoed their stance: "They're fussy, the kids; they eat the cereals, you know, like Coco Pops® and Nutrigrain®" (Warin et al. 2017, pp. 223–224). Another mother told us how her son was very discerning with foods and "won't eat anything if it is past the 'best before' date. So if I go to shop at Rite Price and bring back all this food that is just past the date, even though it's fine, he won't eat it. So I've given up on that. I'm not going to spend my money and have it go to waste. It is just easier and cheaper to get what he'll eat in the first place. He is a real pain in the arse, he is."

People economized on food using a range of strategies: by buying cheaper options, food that is out of date or past the "best before" date, simply buying what they knew would be eaten and fill stomachs rather than unappetizing, healthy foods, purchasing foods with long shelf lives, or omitting meals altogether. Often, the option of sugary cereals or high-fat foods was the easiest, allowing a mother to buy herself time, "five minutes of peace" in the mornings, literally and figuratively sweetening the moment and enabling her to manage her household and cope with its continuous stress. As Berlant (2011) argues, economic threats to families tend to produce households in which "food is one of the few stress relievers" (2011, p. 116) and the eating of sweet foods provides a moment of comfort between children and parents (Warin et al. 2015).

Breaking the Cycle: "It's Not Just Food"

Many of the creative examples of food provision that we observed in people's homes and everyday environments were short-term, creative measures to make ends meet. These are important strategies, but in thinking about sustainable practices, they need to be supported with broader structural measures. In their description of the food bank system in Australia, Booth and Whelan take umbrage with the food bank industry, which implies that the issue of food insecurity is one of "simply needing to have more food available in the pantry" (Booth and Whelan 2014, p. 1400). Having food in the pantry is important, but this will not solve the problem of food poverty. Nor will it address the structural drivers that have given rise to food insecurity, or the rights of people to have the capacity to provide for themselves and their families.

Some participants in our study did talk about long-term strategies to address food poverty and hunger. In a quiet moment in the food bank early on in our fieldwork, Jan told Tanya about her upbringing, going to the computer to show her Facebook photos of her daughter's wedding and her grandchildren. "These are my daughters at my daughter's wedding last year. Don't they look beautiful?" she said, looking proudly at her two girls. She then found a picture of one of her grandchildren. As much as she loves her grandchildren, she is glad when they go home, as she has other caring commitments to attend to. Jan lives with her husband and her elderly father, who has degenerative eye disease and is "pretty much blind." One of the first things that she was eager to tell Tanya about herself was her life trajectory and how she felt she had "broken the cycle." Jan was a single mother on a pension for 20 years before she went back to school and did her final year of study with one of her daughters. After high school she continued with further studies at a Technical and Further Education (TAFE) college, enabling her to gain employment at an adult education campus working with single mums who had returned to studies. "I got a lot of joy out of that. I've a real lot of time for them. They broke the cycle. They never had to, but they did. There are a lot of people out here who've never worked a day in their lives. Dole bludgers,[4] you know? I'm sorry to say it but there are people out there who are just not trying."

Like Yvette, Jan sees herself as an educator. She is proud of these women who were in a position similar to hers, who have "broken the cycle" as she puts it, and are helping themselves financially. "My whole life," she says, "even though I am overweight myself, is based around educating others. Like I was teaching [in adult education] for ten years before I came here [to the food bank], and once again we're trying to break the cycle." She says that means trying to increase awareness about food so people can help themselves. "But," she says, "it's just not food." She describes young mothers who saw their mothers married at 16 years of age: "Well, [their mothers] had babies at 16," and then the daughters thought it "was OK for *them* [emphasis added] to have a baby at 16" and so the pattern is repeated. She sees it as a win if only one of those girls does not follow in her mum's footsteps, but instead finishes school and goes to university: "That's what we're all about here."

Education and employment are key to Jan's pride. Being a working mother, being an example to others, and mentoring are all pursuits that she sees as important. She takes pride in the fact that her children have been educated, have jobs, and are in secure relationships. This is more important than making meals and having a cupboard stocked with food for the short term—this is long-term structural change that underpins people's capacity to have choices, make changes in their everyday lives, and plan for the future.

A key stakeholder in the community spoke to us about the challenge of running an obesity prevention intervention like OPAL. This middle-aged man had worked in the community for many years; he was deeply familiar with community politics and working with local, state, and federal governments. He recounted how difficult it was to create an attitudinal shift in service providers in the direction of preventive health. He could see that OPAL had the opportunity to support a wholesale preventive health agenda that could lead to community regeneration. For him, this wasn't about focusing on healthy eating and weight reduction, but shifting the focus to preventive health measures that meshed with learning and employment pathways. "This," he said, "requires an evolution of thinking in local governments away from the short term, to not think about the last year only but to think long term in a holistic way: to think where have we come from and where are we going? I'm not so much interested in obesity; for me it is about education and employment."

In this chapter we have followed the ways in which stigma, shame, and pride intersect with everyday lives and poverty. We argued that the community has a long history of being stigmatized by outsiders, and that the intersections of working poor, unemployment, and poor health were layered with another level of obesity shame. This was not done overtly, and OPAL was sensitive to the prevailing understanding of stigma in taking care not to impose negative value judgments about the size of large bodies. But obesity stigma is so entrenched in society that it is virtually impossible to erase.

Poor health in this community attracts many judgments about lack of care of self and lack of care of others. OPAL was in the community because of people's BMI scores, and within the community there were judgments made about differing levels of fatness. Some participants were ashamed of others' behaviors (scrounging for cheap and free foods), and made comparisons to distance themselves as "not that bad." Many others took pride in their creative strategies to feed themselves and their households, proud of the fact that they could make ends meet. And others milked the system for what it was worth, getting free handouts from OPAL or performing to the welfare agencies to avoid the endless bureaucratic hoops.

For those people in the community who lived difficult and highly precarious lives, the food bank was a welcoming space to spend divvies on a sweet treat or make the bones of a meal. "Living poor" illustrates what is possible within the constraints of short horizons: it details the improvisations that people make to deal with living presents, rather than anticipated futures. It is a practical realism about the future that is engendered by the reality of the present (Jenkins 2002, p. 28). Importantly, it involves a "taste of necessity" in which survival, and not health, is the priority in many people's lives.

Notes

1. Interestingly, several studies point to different strategies to diminish the stigmatizing impacts of the language of obesity. Vartanian (2010), for example, suggests that using the word fat, rather than obese, results in less stigma. Thomas et al. (2008) also found that people who are overweight or obese prefer the word fat.
2. Megan Carney (2015) makes a similar observation in her ethnographic work on chronic food insecurity among migrant Mexican and Central American women living in Southern California. Participants in her study described "making do" practices, where food and other necessities were limited, rationed, and economized (2015, pp. 169–173).
3. Jack Monroe comes from an English working-class background and found herself unemployed with £10 a week to feed herself and her young son following the global financial crisis and welfare cutbacks. She set about to tackle her own food insecurity, cobbling together ingredients in her tiny kitchen and posting her "austerity recipes" on a blog. She soon became a well-known figure, writing cookbooks (*Cooking on a Bootstrap*, 2018), doing media interviews, and advocating for the rights of people living in poverty. In effect, the "girl called Jack" became the voice of resistance and the face of resilience in austerity Britain.
4. Dole bludger is Australian slang for someone who would rather receive welfare than work. It is a derogatory term replete with negative moral judgments.

References

Adair, V. C. (2002). Branded with infamy: Inscriptions of poverty and class in the United States. *Signs: Journal of Women in Culture and Society, 27*(2), 451–471.

Backett-Milburn, K. C., Wills, W. J., Roberts, M. L., & Lawton, J. (2010). Food, eating and taste: Parents' perspectives on the making of the middle class teenager. *Social Science & Medicine, 71*(7), 1316–1323.

Berlant, L. (2011). *Cruel optimism*. Durham: Duke University Press.

Bombak, A. E., McPhail, D., & Ward, P. (2016). Reproducing stigma: Interpreting "overweight" and "obese" women's experiences of weight-based discrimination in reproductive healthcare. *Social Science & Medicine, 166*, 94–101.

Booth, S., & Whelan, J. (2014). Hungry for change: The food banking industry in Australia. *British Food Journal, 116*(9), 1392–1404.

Bourdieu, P. (2000). *Pascalian meditations* (trans: Nice, R.). Stanford: Stanford University Press.

Braziel, J., & LeBesco, K. (Eds.). (2001). *Bodies out of bounds: Fatness and transgression*. Berkeley: University of California Press.

Brewis, A., Trainer, S., Han, S., & Wutich, A. (2017). Publically misfitting: Extreme weight and the everyday production and reinforcement of felt stigma. *Medical Anthropology Quarterly, 31*(2), 257–276.

Caplan, P. (2016). Big society or broken society?: Food banks in the UK. *Anthropology Today, 32*(1), 5–9.

Carey, G., Malbon, E., Crammond, B., Pescud, M., & Baker, P. (2017). Can the sociology of social problems help us to understand and manage "lifestyle drift"? *Health Promotion International, 32*, 755–761.

Carney, M. A. (2015). *The unending hunger: Tracing women and food insecurity across borders*. Oakland: University of California Press.

Carter, S., Entwistle, V., McCaffery, K., & Rychetnik, L. (2011). Shared health governance: The potential danger of oppressive 'healthism'. *The American Journal of Bioethics, 11*(7), 57–58.

Cooper, C. (2017). *Headless fatties*, Charlotte Cooper website. Available at http://charlottecooper.net/publishing/digital/headless-fatties-01-07

Derrida, J. (1976). *Of Grammatology* (trans: Gayatri Chakravorty Spivak). Baltimore: The Johns Hopkins University Press.

Dobson, B., Beardsworth, A., & Keil, T. (1994). *Eating on a low income*. York: Joseph Rowntree Foundation.

Douglas, F., Sapko, J., Kiezebrink, K., & Kyle, J. (2015). Resourcefulness, desperation, shame, gratitude and powerlessness: Common themes emerging from a study of food bank use in Northeast Scotland. *AIMS Public Health, 2*(3), 297–317.

Dowler, E. (1997). Budgeting for food on a low income in the UK: The case of lone-parent families. *Food Policy, 22*(5), 405–417.

Evans, B., Colls, R., & Hörschelmann, K. (2011). 'Change4Life for your kids': Embodied collectives and public health pedagogy. *Sport, Education and Society, 16*(3), 323–341.

Farrell, A. E. (2011). *Fat shame: Stigma and the fat body in American culture.* New York: New York University Press.

Farrell, L. C., Warin, M., Moore, V. M., & Street, J. M. (2016). Socio-economic divergence in public opinions about preventive obesity regulations: Is the purpose to 'make some things cheaper, more affordable' or to 'help them get over their own ignorance'? *Social Science and Medicine, 154*, 1–8.

Farrugia, D. (2011). The symbolic burden of homelessness: Towards a theory of youth homelessness as embodied subjectivity. *Journal of Sociology, 47*(1), 71–87.

Garthwaite, K. (2016). *Hunger pains: Life inside foodbank Britain.* Bristol: Policy Press.

Garthwaite, K., Collins, P., & Bambra, C. (2015). Food for thought: An ethnographic study of negotiating ill health and food insecurity in a UK foodbank. *Social Science & Medicine, 132*, 38–44. https://doi.org/10.1016/j.socscimed.2015.03.019.

Goffman, E. (1963/2009). *Stigma: Notes on the management of spoiled identity.* New York: Simon and Schuster.

Graham, H., Inskip, H. M., Francis, B., & Harman, J. (2006). Pathways of disadvantage and smoking careers: Evidence and policy implications. *Journal of Epidemiology and Community Health, 60*(2), 7–12.

Green, T., Owen, J., Curtis, P., Smith, G., Ward, P., & Fisher, P. (2009). Making healthy families? In P. Jackson (Ed.), *Changing families, changing food* (pp. 205–225). London: Palgrave Macmillan.

Grosz, E. (1995). *Space, time and perversion: The politics of bodies.* St Leonards/Sydney: Allen and Unwin.

Gunson, J. S., Warin, M., Zivkovic, T., & Moore, V. (2016). Participant observation in obesity research with children: Striated and smooth spaces. *Children's Geographies, 14*(1), 20–34.

Gunson, J. S., Warin, M., & Moore, V. (2017). Visceral politics: Obesity and children's embodied experiences of food and hunger. *Critical Public Health, 27*(4), 407–418.

Guthman, J. (2009). Neoliberalism and the constitution of contemporary bodies. In E. D. Rothblum & S. Solovay (Eds.), *The fat studies reader* (pp. 187–196). New York: New York University Press.

Holmes, M. (2006). Book review: *Blush: Faces of shame*, by Elspeth Probyn. *Body & Society, 12*(1), 123–126.

Jenkins, R. (2002). *Pierre Bourdieu.* London: Routledge.

Lambie-Mumford, H. (2018). 'Every town should have one': Emergency food banking in the UK. *Critical Social Policy*. https://doi.org/10.1177/0261018318765855.

Lister, R. (2004). *Poverty*. Cambridge: Polity.

Lock, M. (1993). *Encounters with aging: Mythologies of menopause in Japan and North America*. Berkeley: University of California Press.

Lupton, D. (2012). *Fat*. London: Routledge.

McCullough, M. (2013). Fat and knocked-up: An embodied analysis of stigma, visibility, and invisibility in the biomedical management of an obese pregnancy. In M. McCullough & A. Hardin (Eds.), *Reconstructing obesity: The meaning of measures and the measures of meanings* (pp. 215–234). New York: Berghahn Books.

McKenzie, L. (2015). *Getting by: Estates, class and culture in austerity Britain*. Bristol: Policy Press.

McRobbie, A. (2005). Notes on 'what not to wear' and post-feminist symbolic violence. In L. Adkins & B. Skeggs (Eds.), *Feminism after Bourdieu* (pp. 99–109). Oxford: Blackwell.

Mol, A., & Law, J. (2004). Embodied action, enacted bodies: The example of hypoglycaemia. *Body & Society, 10*(2–3), 43–62.

Murray, S. (2005). (Un/be)coming out? Rethinking fat politics. *Social Semiotics, 15*(2), 153–163.

Murray, S. (2007). Corporeal knowledges and deviant bodies: Perceiving the fat body. *Social Semiotics, 17*(3), 361–373.

Murray, S. (2008). *The 'fat' female body*. New York: Palgrave.

Pausé, C. (2017). Borderline: The ethics of fat stigma in public health. *The Journal of Law, Medicine & Ethics, 45*(4), 510–517.

Peacock, M., Bissell, P., & Owen, J. (2014). Shaming encounters: Reflections on contemporary understandings of social inequality and health. *Sociology, 48*(2), 387–402.

Peel, M. (1995). *Good times, hard times: The past and the future in Elizabeth*. Carlton: University of Melbourne.

Peel, M. (2004). Imperfect bodies of the poor. *Griffith Review, 4*, 83–93.

Piggin, J., & Lee, J. (2011). 'Don't mention obesity': Contradictions and tensions in the UK Change4Life health promotion campaign. *Journal of Health Psychology, 16*(8), 1151–1164.

Probyn, E. (2005). *Blush: Faces of shame*. Minneapolis: University of Minnesota Press.

Puhl, R. M., & Heurer, C. (2010). Obesity stigma: Important considerations for public health. *American Journal of Public Health, 100*(6), 1019–1028.

Rich, E., De Pian, L., & Francombe-Webb, J. (2015). Physical cultures of stigmatisation: Health policy & social class. *Sociological Research Online, 20*(2), 1–14.

Saguy, A., & Ward, M. (2011). Coming our as fat: Rethinking stigma. *Social Psychology Quarterly, 74*(1), 53–75.

Sayer, A. (2005). *The moral significance of class*. Cambridge: Cambridge University Press.

Scott, J. C. (1985/2008). *Weapons of the weak: Everyday forms of peasant resistance*. New Haven: Yale University Press.

Sennett, R., & Cobb, J. (1972). *The hidden injuries of class*. New York: Vintage.

Shildrick, T., MacDonald, R., Webster, C., & Garthwaite, K. (2010). *The low-pay, no-pay cycle: Understanding recurrent poverty*. York: Joseph Rowntree Foundation.

Thomas, S. L., Hyde, J., Karunaratne, A., Herbert, D., & Komesaroff, P. A. (2008). Being 'fat' in today's world: A qualitative study of the lived experiences of people with obesity in Australia. *Health Expectations, 11*(4), 321–330.

Throsby, K., & Gimlin, D. (2010). Critiquing thinness and wanting to be thin. In R. Ryan-Flood & R. Gill (Eds.), *Secrecy and silence in the research process: Feminist reflections* (pp. 105–116). London: Routledge.

Tyler, I. (2015). Classificatory struggles: Class, culture and inequality in neoliberal times. *The Sociological Review, 63*(2), 493–511.

Vartanian, L. R. (2010). "Obese people" vs. "Fat people": Impact of group label on weight bias, eating and weight disorders. *Studies on Anorexia, Bulimia and Obesity, 15*(3), e195–e198.

Warin, M. J., & Gunson, J. S. (2013). The weight of the word: Knowing silences in obesity research. *Qualitative Health Research, 23*(12), 1686–1696.

Warin, M., Zivkovic, T., Moore, V., Ward, P. R., & Jones, M. (2015). Short horizons and obesity futures: Disjunctures between public health interventions and everyday temporalities. *Social Science & Medicine, 128*, 309–315.

Warin, M., Zivkovic, T., Moore, V., & Ward, P. (2017). Moral fibre: Breakfast as a symbol of a 'good start' in an Australian obesity intervention. *Medical Anthropology: Cross-Cultural Studies in Health and Illness, 36*(3), 217–230.

CHAPTER 8

Conclusion

As we write this conclusion we have just finalized a submission to the Australian Government's Senate Inquiry into the "obesity epidemic in Australia" (July 2018), and appeared in person to give evidence. The 150 written submissions from across Australia represent the range of voices that make this such a political issue—the fast food industry, sugarcane growers in Queensland, university research centers (public health, medicine, and sports), and a number of individual submissions from concerned members of the public. All raise concerns about the "obesity epidemic" and how it should/could be addressed. Australia currently has no national strategy or policy to address obesity, despite the Australian Government highlighting obesity as a problem for at least two decades. There have been many attempts to address healthy eating and activity, but sustained investment in public health programs has been ad hoc and tied to changing government and industry agendas. In our submission we noted the dominant understanding of obesity as a failure of individuals to take responsibility for their own health, and the subsequent failure of behavioral approaches.

An outspoken conservative politician recently weighed in to the national debate over the public pressure to introduce a sugar tax in Australia, suggesting that people need to simply stop eating too much or, failing that, explore options for gastric surgery. George Christensen publicly shared his own experiences of weight loss, traveling to Malaysia for gastric surgery to

M. Warin, T. Zivkovic, *Fatness, Obesity, and Disadvantage in the Australian Suburbs*,
https://doi.org/10.1007/978-3-030-01009-6_8

reduce his body size by half. "The surgery," it was reported, "was a desperate attempt to return to 'good health' and 'not cause a by-election'" (ABC News 2017). Ninety-five percent of Australia's raw sugar is grown in the state of Queensland, and the federal seat of Dawson (George Christensen's electorate) is one of the main centers of the Australian sugar industry.

No one is surprised that Christensen does not support a sugar tax and takes a neoliberal view about obesity. In late 2017 the *New York Times* took an interest in Christensen and the sugar tax debate, producing a short documentary entitled *Do Australians need a sugar intervention?* The documentary includes interviews with Australian media and in it Christensen projects himself as a living example of evidence that the only person to blame for obesity is yourself:

> *I'm a fat bloke, right. I've been fat ever since I was about 20 or 21. But I made poor choices. It wasn't the food industry pushing things down my throat. It was me and the fork or the spoon that I had in my hand. I don't blame the sugar industry. I don't blame Coca Cola. I don't blame XXXX [beer] or Bundaberg Rum, or the residential college that I lived in that had a lot of good food that I liked too, or the servo up the road that served the Chiko Rolls that I liked. I don't blame them. I blame myself for putting that product down my gob. That's what caused it. Me, myself and I. And I think that a lot of the issue with obesity has got to come back to telling people that they are personally responsible for the choices they make.* (ABC 2018)

This causal narrative represents the common-sense approach to understanding obesity, and to a simplistic solution. People should realize that this form of "self-talk" does not constitute research or evidence in the obesity debate; it is just that, one person's experience standing in for everyone's experience. Representing Australia's largest sugarcane-growing industry, it is in Christensen's political interests to support the industry (and vice versa) by promoting "a simple narrative and placing responsibility on consumers to change their behaviour" (Kelly and Russo 2018).

This simplistic understanding of obesity fails at many levels. It fixes fat and blame to individual bodies and fails to understand that food and eating are situated in social practices, and that these practices are relational. People can have excellent knowledge or access to information about nutrition and healthy lifestyles, but this is only one aspect of the myriad of social practices that surround food and eating. Christensen's viewpoint fails to take account of the inequitable distribution of health and disease in our society, and the different circumstances in which people live out their lives. What works for one individual in one location probably won't work for another in a different place. Biologies are local but, as Yates-Doerr reminds us, they can also be contingent and heterogeneous *within* locations (2017, p. 395).[1]

There is overwhelming evidence about the social gradient of obesity in Australia and internationally. Stripping interventions back to individual behavior and bodies does not account for these differences. Obesity Prevention and Lifestyle (OPAL) attempted to move beyond individual blame in its socioecological approach, but we have questioned how this was translated into community initiatives. When we wrote about participants using sweet foods as providing immediate pleasure to ease "things that get under their skin," an OPAL manager said: "But everyone likes chocolate, so what's different here?" Max could acknowledge the relationship between obesity and disadvantage, but could not understand how the value of "enactments of sweetness" could be heightened for those experiencing disadvantage. He found it difficult to see sweetness through the lens of class; as a self-medicating pleasure, the temporal joy of sweetness in lives that had short horizons, and the importance of sweetening relationships (Zivkovic et al. 2015; Warin et al. 2015). The practices of care, sweetness, and pleasure (what Bissell et al. (2016) refer to as "discordant pleasures") were far more important than the *dictum* to cut back sugar and discipline one's body in order to mitigate future health risks.

If we fail to understand the social gradient of obesity within local contexts, then we fail to understand class and the structural conditions of inequality. Moreover, we will continue to see socially undifferentiated messages being directed at people deemed to be too fat. And then we are back at square one.

Class underpinned *all relations* in our fieldwork and informed bodily dispositions of all participants. Middle-class imperatives worked to reshape obese, working-class bodies and families, unfolding a sequelae of class struggles. Class was present in performances of and resistance to normative judgments of "proper" and nutritious eating, was embodied through place and the dynamics of pride and shame, unspoken through the distinction of thinness, and demonstrated via the cultural capital of education and knowledge. These classed contexts produced points of strain and conflict between OPAL workers and some community members, and, in turn, by identifying the politics of class struggles we encountered tensions with our external partners. Class, like the sticky toffee wrapping an apple, became a sticking point in our research relationships.

Seats at the Table

What then, is the role of anthropology in the obesity debate? And why hasn't ethnographic insight generated more value? Why does anthropological knowledge not stick to narratives on obesity? Why is this knowledge devalued in the stakes of what counts? At the OPAL Scientific Committee there were no invited social scientists at the table. An OPAL evaluation manager, who had a background in gender studies, noticed this omission and set up two meetings for a small group of social scientists to meet at different times, at a much smaller table. Ulijaszek (2015) makes the same observations about the UK project Foresight Obesities. Its purpose was to broaden the explanatory frame of obesity studies, but only within bounds, as certain voices were excluded:

> *Foresight Obesities did not encourage critique of the obesity epidemic* (Gard and Wright 2005), *nor did it examine values and norms surrounding large body size, including blame and stigma* (Puhl and Heuer 2009). *These caveats were imposed primarily by choosing carefully who, among the hundreds of experts in the UK, would be invited to participate. Certain challenges in understanding obesity and its drivers were not engaged with, largely by excluding certain types of scholars, especially those that critique the notion of an obesity epidemic or engage with values and norms surrounding body size.*

Ulijaszek concluded that "key experts to the project showed a bias against critical social science approaches to obesity" (2015, p. 218; 2017, p. 177).

Obesity is a highly political issue. From their own ethnographic work, Sanabria and Yates-Doerr reiterate "how experiences of eating and nourishment are embroiled within institutional settings and their attendant knowledge—or non-knowledge—practice" (Sanabria and Yates-Doerr 2015, p. 118; Sanabria 2016). In our research project and our interactions with OPAL and other external partners, we all came to the table with an assumed mutual understanding of obesity and the urgency with which many governments around the world have sought to address it. In many ways this shared footing was necessary and essential for the success of the grant. There was a common ground but it also became the place where uncertainty unfolded. It was extremely difficult while undertaking the research to articulate the ways in which the OPAL team were wedded to a "mode of intervening that has limited purchase on the complexity with which it contends" (Sanabria 2016, p. 154). It was this inability to reorientate the force of prepackaged knowing that became highly problematic.

As we outlined in Chap. 2, for many decades social scientists have offered valuable critiques of medicine and the social construction of disease. We have carved our intellectual space around meaning, experience, and interpretation, adding multiple strands of lay knowledge to the body. The problem with this—as we noted earlier—is that anthropologists (and social scientists) have created a chasm in perspectives about obesity and, in doing so, "granted biomedicine the exclusive right to talk about the body and its diseases" (Mol 2002, p. 13). This has created a stock of knowledge with supporting actors and technologies (body mass index [BMI], apps, body scans, functional foods) continually enrolled into the dominant mode of thinking, thus bolstering taken-for-granted ideas about obesity. This makes it extremely difficult to unsettle the dominant framework of knowing obesity: it must be a problem caused by too much food and too little exercise. Guthman argues that this "energy balance" model is so paradigmatic that to challenge it inevitably raises eyebrows (2012, p. 952).

We have also made important contributions through our fine-grained ethnographic work to understand experiences, local knowledge, and the cultural differences that underpin behaviors. This layering of cultural values is viewed a bit like a recipe to make a cake. It's the "add culture and stir" method. But there are all manner of separate ingredients, of which anthropological knowledge is one, adding taste (both in terms of classed appreciation of foods and pleasure) to the complexity of the cake. In the hierarchical ordering of knowledge, ethnographic insights are layered on top of the biological base, and yet each component remains separate and contained. In this formulation the biological and the social still remain bounded entities.

In OPAL's socioecological approach it was thought that changes to the environment would enable people to attend to behavior change. As we have argued, this well-intentioned attention to the environments in which people are situated was most welcome, but a lifestyle drift back to behaviors meant that the body became the site of what Guthman calls the "socioecological fix" (2015, p. 2523). Situating fat in a classed framework was seen as unpalatable, as was using words from participants that described their own neighborhood or bodies in less salubrious terms.

To describe fat as anything other than associated with ill-health—as positive or useful—was outside the scope of OPAL. Perhaps it was our failure to not articulate clearly enough alternative versions of fatness and obesity—that they could be seen as enactments of abundance. It was telling, at the end of a back and forth negotiation over an academic publication on fatness (with Poppy and our external partners), that these partners were unable to disentangle their equation of fat = ill-health. In an email to the authors expressing their dissatisfaction with our interpretation of fatness, they presented the dominant, singular ontology of fat, writing that

> *[t]here needs to be recognition in the conclusion at least … that fatness is still one of the leading risk factors for the development of many chronic health diseases/conditions. The paper needs to recognize this conundrum.*

What we found in the field, from our interactions with the OPAL program and participants in our research, was that obesity was not one thing, but many things. Obesity was presented as a disease, an epidemic, a problem, caused by a lack of education and lack of knowledge about the right things to eat. What was needed was prescriptions—information about better choices—what to eat and how to exercise. This prescriptive approach to obesity is also seen in the UK, where general practitioners (GPs) may prescribe exercise to obese patients. Obese people are viewed as "fatter than average," and all attempts point toward reducing the negative health effects of too much fat.

For people involved in our study, however, there were multiple versions of obesity and fat was not always "waste" or "matter out of place" (Douglas 1966). People made "agential cuts" (Barad 2007) between enactments of obesity, fat, and fatness. Fatness could be a buffer against the hard knocks of life, a means to keep warm when electricity and gas bills were too expensive; it could be an amalgam of many different drugs and states of being, such as antidepressants, depression, or anxieties. Sweet and fatty foods were not always seen as bad. Sometimes they were necessary supports to relationships of care and to feeling good about oneself. There were many representations of obesity just as there were many versions of fatness (Zivkovic et al. 2018).

These different understandings of fatness or obesity could be present in the same fieldwork spaces—not kept in separate compartments, but constantly circulating, comingling, and clashing. In the food banks people's actions and words around fat, fatness, and obesity appeared and disappeared depending on who was in earshot and which activities were going on. Volunteers and salaried staff could quite happily work at an OPAL local community event and espouse the virtues of sugar-reduced yogurt and healthy smoothies, but did not necessarily practice these eating behaviors themselves. Like the different actors in Mosse's work on development in India, those on the receiving end of a program "create everyday spheres of action autonomous from the organizing policy models (in the manner of de Certeau's analysis), but at the same time work actively to sustain those same models—the dominant interpretations—because it is in their interest to do so" (Mosse 2005, p. 10).

In Chap. 1 we cited Ingold's book (2017) *Knowing from the Inside*, in which he writes: "Sometimes one's best ideas come not from following the main lines of an investigation but from veering off course, in brief encounters with things … and people that trigger reflections on quite unfamiliar and unexpected topics" (2017, p. 4). Conventional obesity interventions come from the outside and use "carrots, sticks, and sermons … to give information and provide facilities such that individuals make 'better' choices for themselves" (Shove et al. 2012, p. 144). Using a practice-oriented approach, we have explored how things came "to be, and hence be known, always and inevitably the result of particular activities and events" (Cohn and Lynch 2017, p. 136). This meant following the ways in which health, bodies, and illness were "made in the context of intimate knowledge about people and their lives" (Yates-Doerr 2015, p. 181).

"What Would You Do?"

"What would you do?" was a question repeatedly asked of us by project partners. What have we learned? Firstly, we have learned that in the current higher education funding environment of impact and engagement ethnographic authority is not enough. Anthropologists are highly skilled in making visible the ways in which knowledge is constructed and then is assumed or taken for granted. We highly value a set of methodological and theoretical skills that "can see through contemporary habits of framing complex conditions" (Sanabria 2016, p. 153). Through our fieldwork in this project we learned about the multiple realities of eating, bodies, and fat, and these realities often seemed contradictory as they shifted through many different contexts in one day (from family homes to OPAL sites, to public spaces). Much of the evidence we provided to our external partners unsettled their existing knowledge, and jarred against the problem that they thought they were addressing. To find that some people were not overly concerned about their body size, that being large afforded certain protections and comforts, that taste and pleasure were more important than nutrients or health, or that nutritionists could themselves be Othered as "skinny Barbie dolls" was discomforting to say the least.

At a time when the OPAL program was undergoing funding cutbacks, we felt there were things we could not say. It was not possible to share our findings from the food banks, as this would have undoubtedly had a disastrous impact on staff and volunteers. Equally, there were findings that could have reflected poorly on OPAL staff, through no fault of their own. We were asked to withhold some of our publications and dissemination until the uncertain political climate changed. The air between us and our external partners became icy and conflict was dealt with by distancing. They wanted to reinforce their expectations, requesting that we conform to council views around a "strengths-based discourse." They wanted us to be enrolled in their project, in their understandings of obesity. Requests were made for a list of our future publications, in attempts to control dissenting interpretations. As Mosse and other critical analysts of policy discourse rightly argue, "[p]ower lies in the narratives that maintain an organization's own definition of the problem—that is, success … depends upon the stabilization of a particular interpretation" (Mosse 2005, p. 8).

If the positioning of local knowledge, practices, and contexts against the dominant paradigm of obesity knowledge is seen as threatening or unwelcome, then how can anthropology engage with these types of problems? How can we bring uncertainty, ambiguity, and instability to a table which is already set?

Luhrmann (2015) offers some practical and wise advice in terms of engaged anthropology. For example, she suggests that all parties should be able to tolerate failures of communication, as it is part of the process of trying to reach out and engage with the world outside of your research group. We would suggest that the same could apply to conflict or points of disagreement. We should not be surprised, when we are dealing with circulations of knowledge, that epistemological conflicts will occur—because epistemologies are always contested. Anthropologists such as Emma Kowal and Eben Kirksey (among others) make this point in their ethnographic writing, noting the multidirectional demands of accountability—from informants who "talk back," from libel laws, from colleagues, and from a reading public who desire particular narrative forms (Kirksey 2009, p. 159; Kowal 2015).

In this ethnography we have presented differing stories and accounts of the practices of obesity and fatness. These are multiple and coexistent realities. As we have shown, these differing versions do not always sit comfortably next to one another, and there is no one knowledge of what obesity is, or how to intervene. Wicked problems cannot be solved with a one-size-fits-all solution. As Law argues, dealing with wicked problems means having the capacity to hold opposites together—"to recognize the [partial] need for homogeneity, centering, closing or dogmatism and even perhaps imperialism … and tempering this with sensitivity to heterogeneity, decentering, openness or lack of dogmatism" (2014, p. 16). The best strategies are likely to be tactical and responsive rather than fixed or large-scale in character—what Law calls "situated forms of interference" (2014, p. 17).

In conclusion, we suggest that a social practice approach to the doing of fatness and obesity can offer some valuable insights into newly imagined health prevention programs. We end by taking a leaf from a very different field, from Indigenous local knowledge practices in Arnhem Land (Northern Territory). In her work on the different and often conflicting, traditional, or science-based practices around land burning, Science and Technology Studies (STS) scholar Helen Verran sought to move beyond "the politics waged over ontic/epistemic commitments" and find ways in which one might do good work—such as negotiating land use—within and between the messiness, contingency, and ineradicable heterogeneity of different knowledge practices (2002). This "situational interference" is what anthropology can offer in the obesity debate, an understanding that scientific approaches to obesity are also a form of traditional knowledge, coming from a canon of Western rationality. If we were to assemble all knowledge practices and compare them, without privileging one over the over, a very useful way may emerge for us to reimagine obesity, and to find new ways to address it.

Note

1. An example of this heterogeneity is provided by Vanessa Agard-Jones in her work on the production of chemical kinships on the pesticide-saturated island of Martinique, where she describes how some bodies can be disproportionately porous (Agard-Jones 2016).

References

ABC. (2017, May 3). Online news report. http://www.abc.net.au/news/2017-05-03/george-christensen-undergoes-radical-weight-loss-surgery/8491884

ABC. (2018). Tipping the scales: Sugar, politics and what's making us fat [television series episode]. In Sarah Ferguson (presenter), *Four Corners*. Sydney: ABC Broadcasting.

Agard-Jones, V. (2016, September 29). CENHS, Episode #35 *Cultures of Energy* [audio podcast]. Retrieved from http://culturesofenergy.com/ep-35-vanessa-agard-jones

Barad, K. (2007). *Meeting the universe halfway: Quantum physics & the entanglement of matter & meaning*. Durham: Duke University Press.

Bissell, P., Peacock, M., Blackburn, J., & Smith, C. (2016). The discordant pleasures of everyday eating: Reflections on the social gradient in obesity under neo-liberalism. *Social Science & Medicine, 159*, 14–21.

Cohn, S., & Lynch, R. (2017). Diverse bodies: The challenge of new theoretical approaches to medical anthropology. *Anthropology & Medicine, 24*(2), 131–141.

Douglas, M. (1966). *Purity and danger: An analysis of the concepts of pollution and taboo*. New York: Pantheon.

Gard, M., & Wright, J. (2005). *The obesity epidemic: Science, morality and ideology*. London: Routledge.

Guthman, J. (2012). Opening up the black box of the body in geographical obesity research: Toward a critical political ecology of fat. *Annals of the Association of American Geographers, 102*(5), 951–957.

Guthman, J. (2015). Binging and purging: Agrofood capitalism and the body as socioecological fix. *Environment and Planning A, 47*(12), 2522–2536.

Ingold, T. (2017). *Knowing from the inside*. Aberdeen: University of Aberdeen.

Kelly, M. P., & Russo, F. (2018). Causal narratives in public health: The difference between mechanisms of aetiology and mechanisms of prevention in non-communicable diseases. *Sociology of Health & Illness, 40*(1), 82–99.

Kirksey, S. E. (2009). Don't use your data as a pillow. In *Anthropology off the shelf: Anthropologists on writing* (pp. 146–159).

Kowal, E. (2015). *Trapped in the gap: Doing good in Indigenous Australia*. Oxford: Berghahn Press.

Law, J. (2014). Working well with wickedness. CRESC (Centre for Research on Socio-Cultural Change) working paper. Retrieved from http://www.cresc.ac.uk/publications/working-well-with-wickedness

Luhrmann, T. (2015). *Making psychological anthropology relevant to global mental health*. [Online video], Society for Psychological Anthropology. Retrieved from https://vimeo.com/145555569

Mol, A. (2002). *The body multiple: Ontology in medical practice*. London: Duke University Press.

Mosse, D. (2005). *Cultivating development: An ethnography of aid policy and practice*. London: Pluto Press.

Puhl, R., & Heuer, C. (2009). The stigma of obesity: A review and update. *Obesity Research, 9*, 788–805.

Sanabria, E. (2016). Circulating ignorance: Complexity and agnogenesis in the obesity epidemic. *Cultural Anthropology, 31*(1), 131–158.

Sanabria, E., & Yates-Doerr, E. (2015). Alimentary uncertainties: From contested evidence to policy. *BioSocieties, 10*, 117–124.

Shove, E., Pantzar, M., & Watson, M. (2012). *The dynamics of social practice: Everyday life and how it changes*. London: Sage.

Ulijaszek, S. (2015). With the benefit of foresight: Reframing the obesity problem as a complex system. *BioSocieties, 10*(2), 213–228.

Ulijaszek, S. J. (2017). *Models of obesity: From ecology to complexity in science and policy*. Cambridge: Cambridge University Press.

Verran, H. (2002). A postcolonial moment in science studies: Alternative firing regimes of environmental scientists and aboriginal landowners. *Social Studies of Science, 32*(5–6), 729–762.

Warin, M., Zivkovic, T., Moore, V., Ward, P., & Jones, M. (2015). Short horizons and obesity futures: Disjunctures between public health interventions and everyday temporalities. *Social Science & Medicine, 128*, 309–315.

Yates-Doerr, E. (2015). *The weight of obesity: Hunger and global health in postwar Guatemala*. Oakland: University of California Press.

Yates-Doerr, E. (2017). Where is the local? Partial biologies, ethnographic sitings. *HAU: Journal of Ethnographic Theory, 7*(2), 377–401.

Zivkovic, T., Warin, M., Moore, V., Ward, P., & Jones, M. (2015). The sweetness of care: Biographies, bodies and place. In L. Attala, E. Abbotts, & A. Lavis (Eds.), *Careful eating: Bodies, food and care* (pp. 109–125). Surrey: Ashgate.

Zivkovic, T., Warin, M., Moore, V., & Ward, P. (2018). Fat as productive: Enactments of fat in an Australian suburb. *Medical Anthropology: Cross-Cultural Studies in Health and Illness, 37*(5), 373–386.

Index[1]

[1] Note: Page numbers followed by 'n' refer to notes.

M. Warin, T. Zivkovic, *Fatness, Obesity, and Disadvantage in the Australian Suburbs*,
https://doi.org/10.1007/978-3-030-01009-6